HISTORY TAKING SKILLS
PHYSICAL EXAMINATION
LABS TEST AND REFERRAL
FOR STUDENTS AND RESIDENTS

HISTORY TAKING SKILLS PHYSICAL EXAMINATION LABS TEST AND REFERRAL FOR STUDENTS AND RESIDENTS

Copyright © 2024 by Huynh Wynn Tran

Cover: Artist Dinh Khai - Book designer: Tien Minh Nguyen

United Buddhist Publisher (UBF)

First printed in California, USA, October 2024

ISBN-13: 979-8-3304-6887-4

© All rights reserved. No part of this book may be reproduced by any means without prior written permission.

HUYNH WYNN TRAN, MD, FACP, FACR

HISTORY TAKING SKILLS PHYSICAL EXAMINATION LABS TEST AND REFERRAL

FOR STUDENTS AND RESIDENTS

UNITED BUDDHIST PUBLISHER

Preface

*Welcome to Wynn Medical Center, where you are about to embark on one of the most important phases of your clinical learning: mastering the **art and science of practicing medicine**. As you join us on this journey, you will become an integral part of our **network of multiple specialty clinics**, all dedicated to delivering **exceptional patient care**.*

This book is designed to guide you through the critical elements of clinical practice, divided into four key parts to provide a comprehensive learning experience:

1. ***History Taking Skills**: Learn the importance of patient interviews, building rapport, and gathering essential clinical information through structured and effective history taking. These skills are fundamental to guiding diagnosis and treatment planning.*
2. ***Physical Examination Skills**: The physical exam is both an art and a science, and mastering it requires careful observation, practice, and attention to detail. This section will take you step-by-step through the techniques needed to perform a thorough and accurate examination.*
3. ***Lab Test Interpretations**: Understanding and interpreting lab results is a key aspect of medical decision-making. This section will equip you with the knowledge to analyze lab findings and integrate them into your clinical reasoning process.*
4. ***When to Refer to a Specialist**: Recognizing when a patient's care requires specialized attention is essential in providing optimal outcomes. This section will help you identify red flags and situations that necessitate referral to specialists, ensuring your patients receive the right care at the right time.*

At Wynn Medical Center, we are committed to fostering an environment of learning and growth. Our multidisciplinary team is here to support you, challenge you, and help you excel in your clinical training.

Huynh Wynn Tran, MD, FACP, FACR
Associate Professor of Medicine and Pharmacy
CEO/Founder of Wynn Medical Center Clinics
Los Angeles, California, USA

CONTENTS

Preface — 5
Part 1: History Taking Skills — 13

- Chapter 1: Foundations of History Taking — 15
  - A. Purpose of History Taking — 15
  - B. Basic Principles — 15
  - C. Ethical Considerations — 17
- Chapter 2: Structure of a Comprehensive History — 19
  - A. Chief Complaint (CC) — 19
  - B. History of Present Illness (HPI) — 19
  - C. Past Medical History (PMH) — 20
  - D. Family History (FH) — 21
  - E. Social History (SH) — 21
  - F. Review of Systems (ROS) — 21
- Chapter 3: Special Situations in History Taking — 22
  - A. Elderly Patients — 23
  - B. Pediatric History — 23
  - C. Obstetric and Gynecologic History — 24
  - D. Psychiatric History — 25
- Chapter 4: Focused History for Specific Complaints — 27
  - A. Cardiovascular History — 27
  - B. Respiratory History — 27
  - C. Gastrointestinal History — 28
  - D. Neurological History — 29
  - E. Musculoskeletal History — 30
- Chapter 5: Improving Communication Skills at Wynn Medical Center — 31
  - A. Building Patient Trust — 31
  - B. Managing Difficult Conversations — 31
  - C. Addressing Cultural Sensitivity — 32
  - D. Language Barriers — 33
- Chapter 6: Common Pitfalls in History Taking — 35
  - A. Biases in History Taking — 35
  - B. Inadequate Listening — 35
  - C. Over-reliance on Technology — 36
- Chapter 7: History Taking in Acute Situations and Telemedicine — 39
  - A. Focused History in Critical Care — 39
  - B. Telephone and Remote History Taking — 40
- Chapter 8: Integrating History Taking with Physical Examination — 43
  - A. Putting Information Together — 43
  - B. Differential Diagnosis Development — 44

Chapter 9: Examples of History Taking of Common Conditions at Wynn Medical Center
- 1. Diabetes Mellitus (Type 2) — 47
- 2. Hyperlipidemia — 47
- 3. Wrist Pain — 48
- 4. Urinary Tract Infection (UTI) — 48
- 5. Psoriasis — 49
- 6. Osteoarthritis — 49
- 7. Chest Pain — 50
- 8. Upper Respiratory Infection (URI) — 50
- 9. Abdominal Pain — 51
- 10. Cervical Radiculopathy — 51
- 11. Low Back Pain — 52

Part 2: The Physical Exam — 53

Chapter 10: Why is the physical exam important? — 55
- A. Role of Physical Examination in Clinical Decision-Making — 55
- B. How to Use This Book — 55
- C. Practical Tips for Integrating Physical Exam Skills into Daily Practice — 56
- D. Common Pitfalls and How to Avoid Them — 56

Chapter 11: General Principles of the Physical Examination — 59
- A. How to Prepare the Patient and the Environment for the Exam — 59
- B. Communication Skills: Explaining the Exam to the Patient — 59
- C. Systematic Approach to the Physical Exam — 60
- D. Infection Control and Hygiene — 60

Chapter 12. Vital Signs and General Appearance — 63
- A. Blood Pressure Measurement Techniques — 63
- B. Pulse, Respiratory Rate, Temperature, and Oxygen Saturation Interpretation — 63
- C. Orthostatic Hypotension Assessment — 64
- E. General Appearance — 65

Chapter 13. Head, Eyes, Ears, Nose, and Throat (HEENT) Examination — 67
- A. Head and Scalp — 67
- B. Eyes — 67
- C. Ears — 68
- D. Nose and Sinuses — 69
- E. Throat and Mouth — 69

Chapter 14. Neck Examination — 71
- A. Thyroid Examination — 71
- B. Lymph Nodes — 71
- C. Jugular Venous Pressure (JVP) — 72

Chapter 15. Cardiovascular Examination — 75
- A. Inspection and Palpation — 75
- B. Auscultation — 75

C. Peripheral Vascular Exam	76
Chapter 16. Respiratory Examination	79
A. Inspection	79
B. Palpation and Percussion	79
C. Auscultation	80
Chapter 17. Gastrointestinal Examination	83
A. Inspection	83
B. Auscultation	83
C. Percussion	83
D. Palpation	84
Chapter 18. Musculoskeletal Examination	87
A. General Inspection	87
B. Joint-Specific Examination	87
C. Spine Examination	88
Chapter 19. Neurological Examination	91
A. Mental Status and Cognitive Function	91
B. Cranial Nerve Examination	91
C. Motor and Sensory Function	92
D. Reflexes	93
E. Coordination and Gait	93
Chapter 20. Dermatologic Examination	95
A. Skin Inspection	95
B. Hair and Nails	96
Chapter 21. Genitourinary Examination	99
A. Male Genitourinary Exam	99
B. Female Genitourinary Exam	99
C. Rectal Examination	100
Chapter 22. Bedside Diagnostic Techniques	103
A. Point-of-Care Ultrasound (POCUS)	103
B. EKG (ECG) Interpretation	103
C. Pulmonary Function Testing (PFTs)	104
Chapter 23. Special Considerations in the Physical Exam	107
A. Elderly Patients	107
B. Obese Patients	107
C. Pediatric Examination	108
Chapter 24. Common Physical Exam Findings and Clinical Correlations at Wynn Medical Center	111
A. Case-Based Learning	111
Heart Failure	111
Cirrhosis	111
Pneumonia	112
Eczema (Atopic Dermatitis)	113

        Chronic Obstructive Pulmonary Disease (COPD)   113

        Type 2 Diabetes Mellitus   114

        Urinary Tract Infection (UTI)   115

        B. Integrating Physical Exam Findings with Diagnostic Work-Up   116

   Chapter 25. Putting All Together: Master the History Taking Skills and Physical Exam at Wynn Medical Center   117

Part 3: Blood Labs and EKG Interpretations   119

   Chapter 26. Common Blood Tests   121

        A. Complete Blood Count   121

        B. Comprehensive Metabolic Panel   123

        C. Urinalysis   125

        D. Lipid Panel   127

        E. Thyroid Panel   129

   Chapter 27. Specialties Blood Test   131

        A. ANA Test   131

        B. ESR/CRP Level   133

        C. Lupus Panel   134

        D. Rheumatoid Arthritis Panel   135

        E. Cancer Markers   136

        F. Vitamin D Level   138

        G. Vitamin B12 Level   140

        H. Hemoglobin A1c and Blood Sugar Level   141

        I. Uric Acid Level   142

   Chapter 28. Other Tests   145

        A. Protein and Urine Electrophoresis   145

        B. Iron Panel   146

        C. Sex Hormones Panel   148

        C. Other Hormones Tests   151

        D. Hepatitis Panel   151

        E. Sexually Transmitted Disease Panel   153

        F. Prostate Panel   154

   Chapter 29. Basic EKG   157

Part 4: When to Refer a Patient to the Specialist?   161

   Chapter 30: General Principles of Referral in Primary Care   163

        A. When to Refer A Patient to A Specialist?   163

        B. Recognizing Red Flags Symptoms Across Systems   164

        C. Balancing Management and Referral   165

   Chapter 31: Cardiovascular Red Flags Symptoms   167

        A. Chest Pain   167

        B. Hypertension   168

        C. Palpitations and Arrhythmias   168

Chapter 32: Respiratory Red Flags Symptoms — 171
- A. Shortness of Breath (Dyspnea) — 171
- B. Cough — 172
- C. Wheezing and Stridor — 173

Chapter 33: Gastrointestinal Red Flags — 175
- A. Abdominal Pain — 175
- B. Dysphagia (Difficulty Swallowing) — 176
- C. Rectal Bleeding — 177

Chapter 34: Neurological Red Flags Symptoms — 179
- A. Headache — 179
- B. Dizziness and Vertigo — 180
- C. Seizures — 180

Chapter 35: Musculoskeletal Red Flags — 183
- A. Back Pain — 183
- B. Joint Pain — 184
- C. Fractures and Trauma — 185

Chapter 36: Endocrine Red Flags Symptoms — 187
- A. Thyroid Disorders — 187
- B. Diabetes — 188
- C. Adrenal Disorders — 188

Chapter 37: Dermatological Red Flags Symptoms — 191
- A. Skin Lesions — 191
- B. Rashes — 192

Chapter 38: Hematological and Oncological Red Flags Symptoms — 195
- A. Anemia — 195
- B. Lymphadenopathy — 196

Chapter 39: Gynecological and Obstetrical Red Flags Symptoms — 199
- A. Pelvic Pain — 199
- B. Abnormal Uterine Bleeding — 200

Chapter 40: Mental Health Red Flags Symptoms — 203
- A. Depression and Suicidality — 203
- B. Psychosis — 204

Chapter 41: Pediatric Red Flags Symptoms — 207
- A. Fever in Infants — 207
- B. Failure to Thrive (FTT) — 208

Part 1: History Taking Skills

Chapter 1: Foundations of History Taking

1.1. Purpose of History Taking

1. **Establishing Trust and Building Patient Rapport**:
    - The medical history is often the first interaction between a clinician and patient, serving as the foundation for building a **therapeutic relationship**. Establishing trust through effective communication fosters **rapport** and encourages patients to share essential information about their health.
    - Research shows that **patients are more likely to disclose sensitive health information** when they feel that their physician is listening empathetically and without judgment. This trust can lead to **improved adherence to treatment plans**, better outcomes, and a more accurate understanding of the patient's condition.
    - Demonstrating respect for the patient's **perspectives** and concerns, acknowledging emotions, and maintaining a non-judgmental stance are key factors in establishing trust early in the patient encounter.
2. **Collecting Key Information to Guide Diagnosis**:
    - The purpose of history taking extends beyond gathering a list of symptoms. It involves **exploring the patient's narrative** and synthesizing the information to guide diagnosis. Studies indicate that a **thorough history accounts for up to 70-90% of accurate diagnoses**, emphasizing its crucial role in clinical practice.
    - By asking structured yet flexible questions, clinicians can identify important details about **the onset, duration, and progression of symptoms**, and detect **red flags** that may indicate serious conditions requiring urgent intervention.
    - Effective history taking also allows clinicians to assess the impact of symptoms on the patient's daily life, providing a holistic view that informs both diagnosis and management.
3. **Creating a Therapeutic Relationship Through Communication**:
    - **Good communication skills** are central to establishing a **therapeutic relationship** with the patient. Clinicians who are able to communicate effectively foster a **collaborative approach** to care, where the patient feels like an active participant in their health management.
    - The **therapeutic relationship** is built on trust, empathy, and clear communication. Through thoughtful, compassionate listening, clinicians can address both **physical** and **psychological concerns**, ensuring that the patient feels heard and valued. A strong therapeutic alliance can enhance treatment adherence and **improve patient satisfaction**.

1.2. Basic Principles

1. **Open-ended vs. Closed-ended Questions**:

- **Open-ended questions** (e.g., "Can you tell me more about your symptoms?") allow patients to provide a narrative, which helps clinicians gather **rich qualitative data** about their symptoms and experiences. This is particularly helpful in understanding **the context of the illness** and its impact on the patient's life .
- **Closed-ended questions** (e.g., "Do you have a fever?") are more focused and elicit **specific answers**, which are useful when confirming details or guiding the conversation in a structured way. A balance of both types is important for thorough history taking .
- A mix of **open and closed questions** ensures that the patient can share their story while allowing the clinician to obtain the necessary clinical details efficiently.

2. **Active Listening and Non-verbal Cues**:
   - **Active listening** involves **full engagement** with the patient during the encounter, reflecting back what the patient says to ensure understanding, and allowing time for the patient to respond. This creates a supportive environment where the patient feels validated .
   - **Non-verbal communication** plays an equally important role. **Body language**, **eye contact**, **nodding**, and **appropriate facial expressions** convey attention and empathy. In fact, studies show that **non-verbal communication** can greatly enhance the patient's perception of the clinician's attentiveness and empathy .
   - **Avoiding distractions**, such as typing on the computer during the patient interview, helps foster a sense of connection and ensures the patient feels listened to.

3. **Ensuring Patient Comfort and Privacy**:
   - Maintaining a **comfortable environment** during history taking is crucial to ensuring the patient feels at ease, which can lead to a more open and honest exchange of information.
   - **Privacy** is particularly important for discussing sensitive issues. Ensuring the room is secure, doors are closed, and unnecessary personnel are excluded helps foster an environment where patients feel comfortable sharing intimate details about their health .
   - **Empathy** and **reassurance** are key when dealing with sensitive or distressing topics. Clinicians should acknowledge the difficulty of discussing certain issues and reassure patients that their concerns will be treated with confidentiality and respect.

4. **Cultural Competence and Addressing Bias**:
   - **Cultural competence** involves understanding and respecting a patient's **cultural beliefs**, values, and practices. It is essential to acknowledge how cultural backgrounds can shape a patient's health behaviors, attitudes toward illness, and expectations from medical care .
   - A culturally competent clinician will adjust their approach to ensure the patient feels respected and understood, which helps **reduce disparities** in healthcare delivery .

- Addressing **implicit bias** is also crucial, as unconscious biases can influence how patients are treated during the history-taking process. **Ongoing self-awareness** and **bias training** are key strategies to mitigate the impact of implicit bias in clinical practice.

1.3. Ethical Considerations

1. **Informed Consent**:
    - **Informed consent** is a cornerstone of ethical medical practice. It ensures that patients are fully informed about their treatment options and the risks/benefits associated with them. During the history-taking process, clinicians should clarify **the purpose of the conversation** and ensure that the patient understands the implications of any diagnostic or therapeutic decisions.
    - In some instances, such as when discussing invasive procedures or sensitive tests, obtaining explicit consent is necessary before proceeding with further evaluation.
2. **Confidentiality and HIPAA Regulations**:
    - **Confidentiality** is a fundamental ethical principle in healthcare. Patients trust that the information they share during a medical history will be **kept private** and protected from unauthorized disclosure. In the U.S., this is reinforced by **HIPAA (Health Insurance Portability and Accountability Act)** regulations, which mandate strict guidelines for safeguarding patient information.
    - Breaching confidentiality can lead to **legal consequences** and a loss of patient trust. Clinicians should ensure that patient data is protected and only shared with relevant healthcare personnel when necessary.
3. **Handling Sensitive Topics with Care**:
    - Discussions about **sexual health, mental illness, substance use**, and **abuse** require a high level of **sensitivity and respect**. When broaching such topics, clinicians should use **empathetic language** and offer reassurance that the information will remain confidential.
    - Techniques like **normalizing the behavior** (e.g., "Many patients struggle with…") can help reduce patient anxiety and foster more open conversations. It is important to be non-judgmental and allow the patient to express their feelings freely without fear of stigma or shame.

References

- Beach, M. C., et al. "Patient-centered communication and diagnostic testing." *Annals of Family Medicine*, 2015.
- Stewart, M. "Effective physician-patient communication and health outcomes: A review." *Canadian Medical Association Journal*, 2019.

- Hampton, J. R., et al. "Relative contributions of history-taking, physical examination, and laboratory investigation to diagnosis and management of medical outpatients." *BMJ*, 2017.
- Levinson, W., et al. "The patient-clinician relationship: the foundation of patient care." *Journal of General Internal Medicine*, 2020.
- Epstein, R. M., et al. "The relationship between physicians' empathy and patients' outcomes." *Journal of General Internal Medicine*, 2018.
- Coulehan, J. L., et al. "Open-ended versus closed-ended questions in eliciting patient symptoms." *Family Practice*, 2016.
- Nunes, P., et al. "Combining open and closed questions in medical consultations." *Journal of Clinical Communication*, 2020.
- Makoul, G., et al. "Essential elements of communication in medical encounters: the Kalamazoo consensus statement." *Academic Medicine*, 2019.
- Hall, J. A., et al. "Non-verbal behavior in clinician-patient interaction: A systematic review." *Journal of General Internal Medicine*, 2018.
- Hojat, M., et al. "The impact of patient confidentiality on patient care." *Medical Ethics Journal*, 2017.
- Betancourt, J. R., et al. "Cultural competence and health care disparities: Key perspectives and trends." *New England Journal of Medicine*, 2019.
- Saha, S., et al. "Cultural competence in health care: A practical guide." *The Lancet*, 2021.
- FitzGerald, C., et al. "Implicit bias in healthcare professionals: a systematic review." *BMC Medical Ethics*, 2020.
- Beauchamp, T. L., et al. "Principles of biomedical ethics." 8th ed., Oxford University Press, 2019.
- U.S. Department of Health and Human Services (HHS). "Summary of the HIPAA Privacy Rule." *HHS.gov*, 2021.
- Lown, B. A., et al. "Handling difficult conversations in medicine: Patient-provider communication strategies." *Journal of Healthcare Communication*, 2020.

Chapter 2: Structure of a Comprehensive History

A comprehensive medical history is the cornerstone of patient assessment and clinical decision-making. It provides vital information that helps guide diagnosis, treatment, and patient management.

A. Chief Complaint (CC)

1. **How to Elicit and Document a Clear Chief Complaint**:
    - The **chief complaint** (CC) is the primary reason the patient is seeking medical care, typically described in one or two sentences. Eliciting a clear chief complaint involves allowing the patient to express their concerns in their own words, ensuring that the physician fully understands the problem.
    - **Open-ended questions** such as "What brings you in today?" encourage patients to describe their symptoms without leading or restricting their responses. This helps clinicians capture the patient's concerns and avoid missing important details.
    - **Documentation** should be concise and use the patient's own words whenever possible. For example, if a patient says, "I have chest pain when I walk," this should be documented verbatim to accurately reflect their experience.
2. **Importance of the Patient's Own Words**:
    - Using the patient's own words ensures that the documentation reflects the true nature of the complaint. It also helps in **rapport building** by validating the patient's concerns. Studies show that documenting the patient's narrative improves **patient satisfaction** and engagement, as they feel heard and understood.

B. History of Present Illness (HPI)

1. **The "OLD CARTS" Mnemonic**:
    - The **HPI** is a detailed account of the patient's symptoms. The **"OLD CARTS" mnemonic** is a helpful tool to guide the clinician in obtaining key information:
        - **O: Onset** – When did the symptom begin?
        - **L: Location** – Where is the symptom located?
        - **D: Duration** – How long has the symptom persisted?
        - **C: Characteristics** – What is the symptom like (sharp, dull, throbbing)?
        - **A: Aggravating and Alleviating factors** – What makes it worse or better?
        - **R: Radiation** – Does the symptom move to other areas?
        - **T: Timing** – Is the symptom constant or intermittent?
        - **S: Severity** – How bad is the symptom on a scale of 1-10?
2. **Chronological Approach to Symptoms**:

- A **chronological approach** allows clinicians to understand the course of the illness. It is helpful to ask the patient to recount their symptoms from the moment they first noticed them to the present, noting any changes or patterns over time. This approach is particularly important in chronic or progressive diseases, such as diabetes or heart failure.
- For example, in the case of chest pain, it is critical to know whether the pain has been intermittent or continuous, how it has evolved, and what previous treatments have been attempted.

3. **Identifying Red Flags in the Patient's History**:
    - **Red flags** are warning signs that suggest potentially serious conditions. For example:
        - In a patient with **chest pain**, red flags might include **shortness of breath**, **diaphoresis**, or **radiation to the left arm**, which could indicate a myocardial infarction.
        - In a patient with **headache**, red flags might include a **sudden onset of severe pain** ("thunderclap headache"), which may suggest a **subarachnoid hemorrhage**.
    - Identifying red flags is essential for triaging patients and prioritizing diagnostic tests and interventions.

C. Past Medical History (PMH)

1. **Common Conditions to Inquire About**:
    - The **PMH** provides insight into a patient's baseline health, comorbidities, and predispositions to certain conditions. Clinicians should ask about common chronic conditions such as **hypertension**, **diabetes**, **heart disease**, **asthma**, and **autoimmune diseases**.
    - **Chronic illnesses** that may have required long-term treatment or hospitalizations, such as **cancer**, **chronic kidney disease**, or **chronic obstructive pulmonary disease (COPD)**, are particularly important to document.

2. **Prior Hospitalizations, Surgeries, and Treatments**:
    - Documenting **previous hospitalizations and surgeries** provides information about the patient's surgical history, complications, and the potential for **postoperative sequelae**. It also highlights any major illnesses or injuries the patient has experienced.
    - Past treatments, including medications or interventions, help in assessing the effectiveness of prior therapies and identifying drug interactions or allergies.

3. **Allergies and Medication Reconciliation**:
    - A thorough review of **allergies** to medications, foods, or environmental factors is critical to avoid adverse reactions. The clinician should inquire about **the type of reaction** (e.g., rash, anaphylaxis) and its severity.

- **Medication reconciliation** ensures that the patient's current medication list is accurate and complete, including **prescription drugs, over-the-counter medications, and supplements**. Incomplete medication histories can lead to **adverse drug interactions** or treatment duplication.

D. Family History (FH)

1. **Key Genetic Conditions and Their Relevance**:
   - Family history provides insight into **genetic predispositions** for certain conditions. Asking about first-degree relatives (parents, siblings, children) with diseases like **heart disease, diabetes, cancer**, or **stroke** is important for assessing **hereditary risk factors**.
   - **Inherited conditions**, such as **cystic fibrosis, sickle cell anemia**, or **Huntington's disease**, should be noted for their potential to affect the patient or offspring.
2. **Focused Questions for Hereditary Diseases**:
   - For patients with suspected genetic predispositions, focused questions should be asked about family members' **age of onset** for conditions like **early-onset heart disease, breast cancer**, or **colorectal cancer**. This information may help guide the need for earlier screenings or genetic counseling.

E. Social History (SH)

1. **Lifestyle Factors**:
   - **Smoking, alcohol, and drug use** are major contributors to disease and are crucial aspects of social history. It is important to quantify use (e.g., **pack-years for smoking, drinks per week for alcohol**) to assess risk for diseases like **lung cancer, cirrhosis**, or **substance use disorders**.
   - Asking about **diet and exercise habits** helps gauge lifestyle factors that may contribute to chronic conditions such as **obesity, hypertension**, and **diabetes**.
2. **Occupational and Environmental Exposures**:
   - **Occupational history** is important for identifying work-related exposures to **toxins, chemicals, dust**, or **repetitive stress** that may lead to diseases such as **occupational asthma** or **mesothelioma**.
   - Environmental exposures, including exposure to **mold, pesticides**, or **air pollution**, can contribute to conditions like **chronic respiratory diseases** and should be explored.
3. **Psychosocial Stressors and Support Systems**:
   - Understanding a patient's **mental health** and **stressors** (e.g., financial hardship, family dynamics) is essential for holistic care. **Depression, anxiety**, and **stress** can exacerbate or trigger physical symptoms and are important to address.

- Assessing a patient's **support systems**, including family, friends, and community resources, is important for understanding the patient's social context and its impact on their health.

F. Review of Systems (ROS)

1. **Systems-based Checklist for Comprehensive History**:
   - The **Review of Systems (ROS)** is a systematic method of inquiring about symptoms related to each organ system. It helps to uncover **hidden symptoms** or **conditions** that the patient may not have initially mentioned.
   - A typical ROS includes **general symptoms** (fever, weight loss), and organ-specific questions (e.g., respiratory symptoms like dyspnea, gastrointestinal symptoms like nausea or vomiting).
2. **Tailoring the ROS to the Patient's Complaint**:
   - The ROS should be tailored to the patient's chief complaint. For example, in a patient presenting with chest pain, the ROS should focus on the **cardiovascular** and **respiratory systems** but should not exclude general symptoms like **fatigue** or **weight changes**, which could provide clues to systemic disease.
   - A targeted ROS can help confirm or rule out differential diagnoses, ensuring that important symptoms are not missed while avoiding irrelevant details that could distract from the primary issue.

References

- McGee, S. "Evidence-Based Physical Diagnosis." 4th ed., Elsevier, 2017.
- Bickley, L. S. "Bates' Guide to Physical Examination and History Taking." 13th ed., Wolters Kluwer, 2021.
- Hampton, J. R., et al. "Relative contributions of history-taking, physical examination, and laboratory investigation to diagnosis and management of medical outpatients." *BMJ*, 2017.
- Smith, R. C., et al. "Patient-centered interviewing: an evidence-based method." 4th ed., Lippincott Williams & Wilkins, 2020.
- Rakel, R. E., et al. "Textbook of Family Medicine." 9th ed., Elsevier, 2020.
- Kempainen, R. R., et al. "Red flags: clinical signs that warrant urgent intervention." *American Journal of Medicine*, 2020.
- Mackenzie, T. A., et al. "Impact of family history on the development of cardiovascular disease: the Framingham Heart Study." *New England Journal of Medicine*, 2021.
- Arnett, D. K., et al. "ACC/AHA Guidelines for Primary Prevention of Cardiovascular Disease: 2019." *Journal of the American College of Cardiology*, 2019.

Chapter 3: Special Situations in History Taking

A. Elderly Patients

1. **Modifying History Taking for Cognitive Impairment**:
   - History taking in elderly patients, particularly those with **cognitive impairment**, requires modifications to ensure accurate and comprehensive information is gathered. **Cognitive decline**, such as **dementia** or **mild cognitive impairment (MCI)**, can affect memory, understanding, and communication, making it necessary to adapt the interview process.
   - Use **short, clear questions** and avoid medical jargon to ensure the patient understands. Incorporating **family members or caregivers** into the history-taking process can provide valuable insights and help fill in gaps in the patient's recollection.
   - Screening for cognitive function using tools like the **Mini-Mental State Examination (MMSE)** or **Montreal Cognitive Assessment (MoCA)** can assist in identifying **cognitive impairment** and guide the approach to history taking.

2. **Identifying Geriatric Syndromes: Falls, Incontinence, Frailty**:
   - **Geriatric syndromes**, including **falls**, **incontinence**, and **frailty**, are common and significantly impact the quality of life in elderly patients. It is important to ask focused questions about these issues during history taking.
     - For **falls**, inquire about recent falls, balance problems, and any injuries. Falls are often multifactorial, related to **muscle weakness**, **medication side effects**, or **vision problems**.
     - For **incontinence**, asking about urinary or fecal leakage and frequency can reveal underlying conditions such as **bladder dysfunction** or **neurological impairment**.
     - **Frailty** refers to a state of decreased physiological reserve, making elderly patients more vulnerable to stressors. **Weight loss**, **fatigue**, and **decreased activity levels** are key indicators of frailty.

3. **Polypharmacy and Medication History**:
   - **Polypharmacy** (the use of multiple medications) is common among elderly patients and increases the risk of **adverse drug reactions**, **drug interactions**, and **medication non-adherence**. A detailed review of all **prescription medications**, **over-the-counter drugs**, and **supplements** is critical.
   - Use tools like the **Beers Criteria** to identify potentially inappropriate medications in older adults. Ask about medication adherence, as **cognitive issues** or **financial constraints** can lead to missed doses or inappropriate medication use.
   - Assess for symptoms that may be caused by medication side effects, such as **dizziness**, **confusion**, or **falls**.

B. Pediatric History

1. **Obtaining History from Caregivers**:
   - In pediatric patients, the **caregiver**, often the parent, is the primary source of information. It is important to build trust with the caregiver and engage them in a way that elicits accurate and complete information about the child's health.
   - Begin with open-ended questions like, "What concerns you the most about your child's health?" and follow up with more specific inquiries. It is also important to **observe the child's behavior** during the history-taking process, as non-verbal cues may provide additional insights.
2. **Developmental Milestones and Immunization Status**:
   - **Developmental history** is crucial for assessing a child's progress and identifying delays early. Ask about **milestones** in areas such as **motor skills**, **language**, **social interaction**, and **cognitive development**. Using standardized screening tools like the **Ages and Stages Questionnaire (ASQ)** can help quantify developmental progress.
   - Immunization status should be reviewed during every visit to ensure the child is up to date according to **CDC immunization schedules**. Missed vaccinations increase the risk of preventable diseases and should be addressed immediately.
3. **Addressing Common Pediatric Concerns (Feeding, Sleep, Behavior)**:
   - Pediatric history should also address common concerns such as **feeding**, **sleep**, and **behavior**. For infants, ask about breastfeeding or formula feeding, the frequency of feeds, and any concerns with **latching** or **weight gain**.
   - For older children, inquire about **sleep patterns**, including **bedtime routines**, **night awakenings**, and the duration and quality of sleep. Sleep disturbances may be related to **anxiety**, **diet**, or **developmental issues**.
   - Behavioral concerns, including **temper tantrums**, **hyperactivity**, or **aggression**, may warrant further evaluation for underlying developmental or psychosocial issues such as **autism spectrum disorder** or **ADHD**.

C. Obstetric and Gynecologic History

1. **Key Aspects of Reproductive History: Pregnancies, Menstrual History, Contraception**:
   - A thorough **obstetric and gynecologic history** should include a review of the patient's **pregnancy history** (number of pregnancies, outcomes, complications), **menstrual history** (age of menarche, regularity, flow, and associated symptoms), and **contraception use**.
   - Ask about the **date of last menstrual period (LMP)** and any **abnormal uterine bleeding**, as these may signal conditions such as **fibroids**, **endometrial hyperplasia**, or **hormonal imbalances**.

- In sexually active patients, explore the use of **contraceptive methods** and discuss the risks and benefits of various options, such as **oral contraceptives**, **IUDs**, or **barrier methods**.
2. **Addressing Sensitive Topics Like Sexual Health, Infertility, and Menopause**:
    - **Sexual health** is an integral part of reproductive history and should be approached with sensitivity. Ask about sexual activity, **STI prevention**, and any **pain** or **discomfort** during intercourse (dyspareunia). Ensure the patient feels comfortable discussing these topics by using non-judgmental, open-ended questions.
    - **Infertility** can be an emotionally charged topic, so it's important to ask about efforts to conceive, duration of infertility, and previous workup or treatments in a compassionate and supportive manner.
    - In peri- and post-menopausal patients, inquire about symptoms related to **menopause** such as **hot flashes**, **vaginal dryness**, and **mood changes**. These symptoms may impact the quality of life and should be addressed as part of holistic care.

D. Psychiatric History

1. **Techniques for Assessing Mental Health Conditions**:
    - Mental health conditions such as **depression**, **anxiety**, and **bipolar disorder** require careful, empathetic history-taking. Begin by asking about **mood** and **emotions** using open-ended questions such as "How have you been feeling lately?" and follow up with more specific inquiries about **sleep**, **appetite**, and **energy levels**.
    - Screening tools like the **Patient Health Questionnaire-9 (PHQ-9)** for depression or the **Generalized Anxiety Disorder 7-item scale (GAD-7)** can be useful to quantify symptoms and gauge severity.
    - Pay attention to **non-verbal cues** such as **affect**, **eye contact**, and **motor activity**, which may provide additional insights into the patient's mental state.
2. **Suicide Risk Assessment and Evaluating Mood Disorders**:
    - **Suicide risk assessment** is a critical component of psychiatric history taking, especially in patients with **depression** or **bipolar disorder**. Asking direct questions such as, "Have you ever thought about hurting yourself?" or "Do you have a plan?" is essential in identifying patients at risk.
    - Evaluate for **protective factors** such as family support, religious beliefs, and personal coping strategies, as these can help mitigate risk. In high-risk cases, **emergency intervention** or referral to psychiatric care may be warranted.
3. **Substance Use History and Motivational Interviewing**:
    - Inquiring about **substance use** (alcohol, tobacco, recreational drugs, prescription drug misuse) should be done in a non-judgmental manner. Use validated tools like **AUDIT (Alcohol Use Disorders Identification Test)** to assess alcohol

consumption, and the **CAGE questionnaire** to screen for problematic drinking behaviors.
- ○ **Motivational interviewing** techniques can help engage patients who are ambivalent about changing their substance use. Asking open-ended questions, affirming the patient's autonomy, and helping them explore the pros and cons of their behavior can facilitate change and promote healthier decisions.

References

- Bickley, L. S. "Bates' Guide to Physical Examination and History Taking." 13th ed., Wolters Kluwer, 2021.
- McGee, S. "Evidence-Based Physical Diagnosis." 4th ed., Elsevier, 2017.
- Tinetti, M. E., et al. "Geriatric syndromes and falls: A critical challenge in managing older adults." *Journal of the American Geriatrics Society*, 2019.
- Hebert, L. E., et al. "Alzheimer's disease in the United States (2010–2050) estimated using the 2010 census." *Neurology*, 2020.
- Squires, J., et al. "Screening for developmental delays: The importance of early detection and intervention." *Journal of Early Childhood Research*, 2018.
- Powers, N. G., et al. "Common pediatric feeding problems: An overview and assessment guide." *Pediatrics*, 2017.
- ACOG Practice Bulletin. "Well-woman visits: Guidelines for reproductive health care." *Obstetrics & Gynecology*, 2018.
- American Psychiatric Association. "Guidelines for suicide risk assessment and management." *APA Practice Guidelines*, 2021.
- Rollnick, S., et al. "Motivational interviewing in health care: Helping patients change behavior." *American Journal of Lifestyle Medicine*, 2019.
- Kroenke, K., et al. "The PHQ-9: Validity of a brief depression severity measure." *Journal of General Internal Medicine*, 2020.

Chapter 4: Focused History for Specific Complaints

A. Cardiovascular History

1. **Chest Pain, Palpitations, Syncope, Dyspnea**:
    - **Chest pain** is one of the most common reasons for seeking medical care and can indicate life-threatening conditions like **myocardial infarction (MI)**, **pulmonary embolism**, or **aortic dissection**. It's important to ask about the **quality, location, radiation**, and **associated symptoms** of the pain. Classic ischemic chest pain is described as **pressure-like, substernal**, and may radiate to the **left arm** or **jaw**.
        - **Red flags**: Acute, crushing pain, particularly with **diaphoresis, nausea**, or **shortness of breath**, warrants immediate evaluation for acute coronary syndrome (ACS).
    - **Palpitations** may indicate arrhythmias, **thyrotoxicosis**, or **anxiety**. Ask about the **onset, duration**, and **frequency** of palpitations, along with associated symptoms like **dizziness** or **syncope**. Palpitations accompanied by **syncope** suggest arrhythmias such as **ventricular tachycardia**.
    - **Syncope** often reflects **cardiac arrhythmias, orthostatic hypotension**, or **vasovagal responses**. It's important to differentiate true syncope (transient loss of consciousness) from **near-syncope** and inquire about **triggers, prodromal symptoms** (e.g., dizziness, nausea), and **recovery**.
    - **Dyspnea** may suggest heart failure, **pulmonary embolism**, or **COPD**. In cardiovascular pathology, dyspnea that worsens with exertion or occurs when lying down (**orthopnea**) is often indicative of **left-sided heart failure**.
2. **Identifying Risk Factors for Coronary Artery Disease and Heart Failure**:
    - **Coronary artery disease (CAD)** and **heart failure** are strongly associated with traditional risk factors, including:
        - **Hypertension**: Chronic high blood pressure increases the workload on the heart.
        - **Diabetes**: Patients with diabetes are at higher risk of developing CAD and heart failure.
        - **Hyperlipidemia**: Elevated **LDL** and low **HDL** cholesterol levels contribute to atherosclerosis.
        - **Smoking**: Strongly associated with both **atherosclerosis** and **heart failure**.
        - **Family history**: A first-degree relative with CAD or heart disease increases a patient's risk of similar conditions.
3. Inquiring about these factors helps stratify risk and guide further diagnostic testing, such as an **electrocardiogram (ECG), echocardiography**, or **stress testing**.

B. Respiratory History

1. **Cough, Wheezing, Hemoptysis, Shortness of Breath:**
    - A **cough** can have multiple etiologies, ranging from benign **upper respiratory tract infections** to serious conditions like **lung cancer** or **tuberculosis**. Ask about the **duration** (acute vs. chronic), the **character of the cough** (productive vs. dry), and any **associated symptoms** (e.g., fever, weight loss).
        - Chronic coughs are often linked to **asthma, COPD, gastroesophageal reflux disease (GERD)**, or **postnasal drip**.
    - **Wheezing** is typically associated with airway obstruction, commonly seen in **asthma** or **COPD**. Ask about **triggers** (e.g., allergens, exercise) and any history of **inhaler use**.
    - **Hemoptysis** (coughing up blood) can be a sign of serious conditions like **lung cancer, tuberculosis**, or **pulmonary embolism**. Clarify whether the blood is mixed with sputum or if it's a pure blood expectoration. Acute hemoptysis warrants immediate investigation.
    - **Shortness of breath** (dyspnea) has both **cardiac** and **pulmonary causes**. Asking about **exertional dyspnea, nocturnal dyspnea**, and any associated chest pain can help distinguish between **heart failure** and **respiratory conditions**.
2. **Occupational and Environmental Exposures:**
    - Occupational and environmental exposures are critical factors in **respiratory disease**. Ask about the patient's occupation (e.g., **mining, farming, construction**) to identify possible exposures to **asbestos, silica**, or **coal dust**, which can cause diseases such as **asbestosis, silicosis**, or **coal worker's pneumoconiosis**.
    - Environmental exposures, such as **smoke, pollution**, or exposure to **mold**, can exacerbate conditions like **asthma** and **COPD**.

C. Gastrointestinal History

1. **Abdominal Pain, Nausea, Vomiting, Diarrhea, Constipation:**
    - **Abdominal pain** can have numerous causes, and the history should focus on the **location, character**, and **timing** of the pain. For example, **right upper quadrant pain** may suggest **cholecystitis**, while **epigastric pain** may point to **peptic ulcer disease** or **pancreatitis**. Pain that worsens after meals may suggest **gallstones** or **intestinal ischemia**.
    - **Nausea and vomiting** may be associated with conditions like **gastroenteritis, bowel obstruction**, or **pancreatitis**. Ask about the **quality** and **timing** of vomiting, as well as any **relationship to meals**.
    - **Diarrhea** can indicate **infectious gastroenteritis, inflammatory bowel disease**, or **malabsorption syndromes**. Ask about the **frequency, consistency**, and **appearance** of the stools, as well as any recent travel or antibiotic use.

- **Constipation** is commonly seen in **functional bowel disorders** or may be secondary to medications such as **opioids** or **iron supplements**. Ask about the **duration**, **stool consistency**, and any associated symptoms such as **pain** or **rectal bleeding**.
2. **Key Questions for Liver, Gallbladder, and Pancreas**:
    - In patients with suspected **liver disease**, ask about **jaundice**, **dark urine**, **pale stools**, and **pruritus**. For chronic liver disease, ask about **alcohol use**, **hepatitis risk factors**, and any history of **liver cirrhosis**.
    - **Gallbladder disease** often presents with **right upper quadrant pain** that radiates to the **right shoulder**, often triggered by fatty meals. Ask about **biliary colic**, **fever**, or signs of **cholangitis** (jaundice, fever, RUQ pain).
    - **Pancreatic disease** typically presents with **epigastric pain** that radiates to the back and worsens after eating. Ask about risk factors such as **alcohol use** and **gallstones**. **Weight loss** and **steatorrhea** (fatty stools) can indicate **pancreatic insufficiency** .

D. Neurological History

1. **Headache, Dizziness, Weakness, Seizures**:
    - **Headaches** require careful characterization. Ask about the **location**, **intensity**, and **quality** (e.g., throbbing, pressure) of the headache. Red flags include **thunderclap onset**, **fever**, **neck stiffness**, and **neurological deficits**, which may suggest conditions like **subarachnoid hemorrhage** or **meningitis** .
    - **Dizziness** can refer to either **vertigo** (a spinning sensation) or **lightheadedness**. Vertigo may indicate **benign paroxysmal positional vertigo (BPPV)**, **Meniere's disease**, or **vestibular neuronitis**. Associated symptoms like **hearing loss** or **tinnitus** can help narrow the differential.
    - **Weakness** requires differentiation between **focal** and **generalized** weakness. Focal weakness (e.g., unilateral limb weakness) suggests **stroke** or **transient ischemic attack (TIA)**, while generalized weakness may indicate **myopathy**, **Guillain-Barré syndrome**, or **myasthenia gravis**.
    - **Seizures** should be characterized by their **duration**, **triggers**, and **associated symptoms**. Ask about a history of **head trauma**, **fever**, or **substance use**. **Postictal confusion** suggests a generalized seizure, while **focal neurological deficits** may suggest a **brain lesion** or **stroke**.
2. **Focal Deficits and Identifying Red Flags for Neurological Emergencies**:
    - Red flags in neurological history include **sudden-onset weakness**, **altered consciousness**, and **loss of coordination**, which may suggest **stroke**, **brain hemorrhage**, or **spinal cord compression**.
    - Early identification of **stroke symptoms** using the **FAST mnemonic** (Face drooping, Arm weakness, Speech difficulty, Time to call 911) is critical for timely intervention .

E. Musculoskeletal History

1. **Joint Pain, Swelling, Stiffness, Injury History**:
   - **Joint pain** may arise from inflammatory or non-inflammatory conditions. Ask about the **onset**, **duration**, and **symmetry** of joint involvement. **Morning stiffness** lasting more than 30 minutes is often seen in inflammatory conditions like **rheumatoid arthritis**, whereas brief stiffness suggests **osteoarthritis**.
   - **Swelling** and **warmth** of a joint suggest active inflammation, which could be caused by **infection**, **gout**, or **rheumatoid arthritis**. A history of trauma or overuse may point to **tendinitis**, **bursitis**, or **ligament injury**.
   - Ask about prior **injuries** or surgeries involving the affected joints, as previous trauma can lead to **degenerative changes** over time.
2. **Identifying Patterns of Autoimmune or Inflammatory Conditions**:
   - Autoimmune diseases like **systemic lupus erythematosus (SLE)**, **psoriatic arthritis**, or **ankylosing spondylitis** often involve **multiple systems**. Ask about **rash**, **eye inflammation**, **GI symptoms**, and **family history** of autoimmune diseases. Morning stiffness, symmetrical joint involvement, and systemic symptoms like fever and fatigue suggest an inflammatory cause.
   - **Back pain** in young adults that is worse at night and improves with activity may indicate **ankylosing spondylitis**. Ask about a family history of autoimmune disorders and any associated symptoms like **uveitis** or **inflammatory bowel disease**.

References

- Bickley, L. S. "Bates' Guide to Physical Examination and History Taking." 13th ed., Wolters Kluwer, 2021.
- McGee, S. "Evidence-Based Physical Diagnosis." 4th ed., Elsevier, 2017.
- Ropper, A. H., et al. "Adams and Victor's Principles of Neurology." 11th ed., McGraw Hill, 2019.
- Williams, B. A., et al. "Evaluating Patients with Acute Chest Pain in the Emergency Department." *JAMA*, 2019.
- Colledge, N. R., et al. "Occupational Exposures and Respiratory Health." *Lancet Respiratory Medicine*, 2020.
- Tinetti, M. E., et al. "Geriatric Syndromes: Clinical, Research, and Policy Implications of a Core Geriatric Concept." *JAMA Internal Medicine*, 2021.
- Shekelle, P., et al. "Management of Chronic Musculoskeletal Pain." *BMJ*, 2020.
- American College of Rheumatology. "Guidelines for the Management of Rheumatoid Arthritis." *ACR Guidelines*, 2021.

Chapter 5: Improving Communication Skills at Wynn Medical Center

Effective communication is the foundation of a successful clinician-patient relationship, fostering trust, empathy, and collaboration.

A. Building Patient Trust

1. **Creating a Supportive Environment**:
    - Building trust with patients begins with creating a **supportive and welcoming environment**. Patients are more likely to share their concerns when they feel **safe and respected**. Research shows that **non-verbal cues** such as maintaining **eye contact**, providing **undivided attention**, and using **open body language** significantly improve trust and rapport .
    - A supportive environment is also created by demonstrating **active listening** and **encouraging patient engagement**. When patients perceive their physician as empathetic and understanding, they feel more confident in discussing their symptoms and concerns openly. This not only enhances trust but also improves **clinical outcomes** .
2. **Empathy and Validation in History Taking**:
    - **Empathy** involves recognizing and acknowledging the patient's feelings, which helps validate their experiences and emotions. A simple statement like, "I understand that this must be difficult for you," can reassure patients that their concerns are taken seriously.
    - Studies show that physicians who practice **empathetic communication** achieve better patient satisfaction, improved adherence to treatment plans, and more accurate diagnoses. Empathy also reduces **patient anxiety** and fosters a sense of partnership in care .
    - **Reflective listening** is an important tool to demonstrate empathy, where the physician repeats or rephrases what the patient has said to ensure clarity and understanding. For example, "It sounds like you've been feeling very tired lately, is that right?"

B. Managing Difficult Conversations

1. **Breaking Bad News**:
    - Breaking bad news requires sensitivity and clarity. The **SPIKES protocol** is a widely used approach that helps structure these conversations:
        - **S**: **Setting** – Ensure privacy, involve family members if appropriate, and minimize distractions.
        - **P**: **Perception** – Assess the patient's understanding of their situation before delivering news.
        - **I**: **Invitation** – Ask the patient how much information they wish to receive.

- **K: Knowledge** – Provide information in small, clear segments, using simple language.
- **E: Empathy** – Acknowledge emotions and offer support.
- **S: Summary and Strategy** – Summarize the conversation and discuss the next steps for care.
    - Physicians should be mindful of **non-verbal cues** and **patient reactions** during these conversations. It's important to pause and allow the patient to process the information, offering emotional support when needed.

2. **Dealing with Non-Compliant Patients**:
    - **Non-compliance** often stems from a lack of understanding, cultural beliefs, or other barriers to care. The first step is to **explore the reasons for non-compliance** in a non-judgmental manner. Open-ended questions such as, "Can you help me understand why taking your medication has been challenging?" can uncover hidden concerns or misconceptions.
    - **Motivational interviewing** is a valuable technique to encourage behavior change. This approach involves helping the patient explore their own reasons for change and emphasizing their autonomy in decision-making. It is particularly useful in chronic disease management, such as **diabetes** or **hypertension**, where long-term adherence is critical.

3. **Handling Angry or Upset Patients**:
    - When dealing with **angry or upset patients**, remaining calm and composed is crucial. Start by acknowledging the patient's feelings, saying something like, "I can see that you're frustrated, and I want to help." This shows that you are listening and ready to address their concerns.
    - **De-escalation techniques** involve using a calm voice, open body language, and active listening to diffuse tension. Asking clarifying questions such as, "Can you tell me more about what's bothering you?" can help redirect the conversation to problem-solving.
    - Sometimes, allowing the patient to vent for a moment can help reduce their emotional intensity. Afterward, focusing on solutions and ensuring follow-up actions can rebuild trust and cooperation.

C. Addressing Cultural Sensitivity

1. **Respecting Diverse Backgrounds and Traditions**:
    - Cultural sensitivity is essential for effective communication, particularly in a diverse patient population. **Cultural competence** involves understanding and respecting patients' cultural backgrounds, values, and health practices. Research has shown that physicians who demonstrate cultural competence can improve patient satisfaction and adherence to treatment.
    - For example, some Vietnamese patients may prefer **alternative medicine** or hold **traditional health beliefs** that differ from conventional medical practices. Rather than dismissing these beliefs, physicians should explore them and work

collaboratively with patients to incorporate safe practices while providing evidence-based care. Statements like, "I understand that this treatment is important in your culture. Let's talk about how we can integrate it with the care I'm providing" can help build trust .

2. **Understanding Health Beliefs and Practices in Different Cultures**:
   - Certain cultural groups may have distinct beliefs about **illness** and **healing**. For example, some cultures may attribute illness to **spiritual causes**, while others may prefer **family-centered decision-making**. Understanding these cultural nuances helps the physician navigate sensitive conversations and respect the patient's preferences .
   - Asking questions such as, "Are there any cultural practices or beliefs I should be aware of when discussing your treatment?" allows the patient to express their values and promotes a more patient-centered approach. Culturally tailored interventions have been shown to improve health outcomes, especially in chronic disease management .

D. Language Barriers

1. **Using Professional Interpreters**:
   - Language barriers can significantly impact communication and patient safety. The use of **professional interpreters** is strongly recommended over relying on family members or untrained individuals, as they ensure accurate translation and maintain confidentiality.
   - Research has shown that using trained interpreters reduces medical errors, increases patient understanding, and improves patient satisfaction. In situations where interpreters are not available in person, **telephonic or video interpretation services** can provide effective alternatives .
   - During conversations with interpreters, it is important to speak directly to the patient rather than the interpreter, maintaining eye contact and engagement with the patient to foster trust.

2. **Avoiding Medical Jargon**:
   - Patients with limited health literacy or non-native speakers may struggle with medical terminology. To ensure understanding, clinicians should **avoid medical jargon** and use **simple, clear language**. For example, instead of saying "hypertension," use "high blood pressure," or instead of "edema," say "swelling."
   - Using the **teach-back method**—asking patients to explain the information in their own words—can help confirm comprehension. Studies show that patients who demonstrate understanding of their condition are more likely to adhere to treatment and experience better outcomes .

3. **Ensuring Clear Communication with Patients**:
   - Clear communication goes beyond language proficiency. It includes **verbal clarity**, **body language**, and ensuring the patient feels comfortable asking

questions. Creating an environment where patients feel empowered to clarify or repeat information can prevent misunderstandings and improve care.
    - Encourage patients to ask questions by saying, "Do you have any questions about what we've discussed?" or "Is there anything you'd like me to explain further?" This opens the door for patients to engage in their care actively.

References

- Beach, M. C., et al. "Patient-centered communication and diagnostic testing." *Annals of Family Medicine*, 2015.
- Levinson, W., et al. "Effective communication in primary care: A key to improved health outcomes." *Journal of General Internal Medicine*, 2020.
- Baile, W. F., et al. "SPIKES—a six-step protocol for delivering bad news: application to the patient with cancer." *The Oncologist*, 2021.
- Rollnick, S., et al. "Motivational interviewing in health care: Helping patients change behavior." *American Journal of Lifestyle Medicine*, 2019.

Chapter 6: Common Pitfalls in History Taking

History taking is a crucial component of clinical practice, but certain pitfalls can impede the process and lead to misdiagnosis or incomplete patient care. Understanding and addressing these common pitfalls is essential for clinicians to improve patient outcomes and ensure accurate diagnoses

A. Biases in History Taking

1. **Avoiding Diagnostic Anchoring**:
   - **Diagnostic anchoring** occurs when a clinician becomes fixated on an initial diagnosis based on early, limited information, leading to **premature closure** in the diagnostic process. Once a clinician anchors on a particular diagnosis, they may disregard new evidence or alternative possibilities.
   - To avoid anchoring, clinicians should remain open-minded throughout the patient interview and be aware of **confirmation bias**, where they seek evidence to support their initial hypothesis while ignoring contradictory data. Research has shown that diagnostic errors are frequently linked to **cognitive biases**, including anchoring, which can be particularly dangerous in complex cases .
   - To mitigate this risk, using a structured approach such as considering a **differential diagnosis** or using the **Socratic method** of questioning (asking what else could explain the symptoms) can help prevent tunnel vision. Encouraging **team-based discussions** where colleagues can provide alternative viewpoints is also beneficial .
2. **Recognizing Implicit Biases**:
   - **Implicit biases** are unconscious attitudes or stereotypes that can affect clinical decision-making. These biases can lead to differential treatment based on factors like **race**, **gender**, **age**, or **socioeconomic status**, often resulting in poorer care for marginalized populations.
   - For example, studies have shown that African American patients are less likely to receive adequate pain management compared to their white counterparts, due in part to implicit biases about pain tolerance .
   - To counter implicit bias, clinicians must engage in **self-reflection** and **bias training**, and integrate practices like **shared decision-making**, which involves the patient in the care process. Bias awareness tools, such as **Harvard's Implicit Association Test (IAT)**, can help clinicians recognize and address their unconscious biases, ensuring more equitable care.

B. Inadequate Listening

1. **Importance of Allowing the Patient to Speak Without Interruption**:
   - Interrupting patients during history taking can lead to incomplete data collection and missed diagnoses. Research has shown that on average, clinicians interrupt

patients **within 11 seconds** of the patient beginning to speak, cutting off valuable information that may guide diagnosis .
- Allowing the patient to express their concerns fully is critical. Patients often provide key details about their symptoms or history in their own narrative, and interruptions can disrupt the flow of vital information. Studies have shown that patients typically complete their initial narrative in less than two minutes when allowed to speak uninterrupted .
- **Active listening**—where the clinician demonstrates attentiveness and gives non-verbal cues to encourage the patient to continue—helps the patient feel heard and builds rapport. Additionally, this approach provides a more complete picture of the patient's condition.

2. **Addressing the "Hidden Agenda"**:
    - Patients often have a **"hidden agenda"**—concerns or issues they don't immediately share during the history-taking process, often because they feel embarrassed, fear judgment, or don't believe it's relevant. Common examples include concerns about **sexual health**, **mental health**, or sensitive social issues.
    - Clinicians can uncover these hidden agendas by using open-ended questions like, "Is there anything else you'd like to talk about today?" or "Are there any concerns that we haven't covered?" These prompts invite patients to share additional information they may have been withholding.
    - Studies suggest that addressing these hidden concerns early in the encounter can reduce **repeat visits** and improve **patient satisfaction**, as the patient feels their concerns were adequately addressed .

C. Over-reliance on Technology

1. **Maintaining the Patient-Centered Focus Despite the Presence of Electronic Medical Records (EMRs)**:
    - **Electronic Medical Records (EMRs)** have become an essential tool in modern healthcare, but an over-reliance on EMRs during history taking can detract from the **patient-centered approach**. Clinicians who spend too much time focusing on the computer screen may inadvertently disengage from the patient, leading to decreased **eye contact**, **non-verbal communication**, and rapport.
    - Research shows that patients perceive physicians who frequently look at the computer during visits as less attentive and empathetic, which can reduce trust and hinder the therapeutic relationship .
    - To avoid over-reliance on technology, clinicians should prioritize **face-to-face interaction** during history taking. One approach is the "three-stage process" for balancing EMR use:
        - **First**, start the consultation with direct patient engagement, listening to the patient's concerns without distraction.
        - **Second**, involve the patient when using the EMR, explaining what you're doing as you type or access records.

- **Third**, conclude with a final period of direct communication, summarizing the key points of the encounter and ensuring that the patient's concerns have been addressed .
    - Using technology to enhance rather than detract from patient interaction—such as turning the screen to show the patient relevant lab results or diagrams—can help maintain a collaborative approach.
2. **Pitfalls of Copy-Pasting in EMRs**:
    - The convenience of **copy-pasting notes** in EMRs can lead to **documentation errors** and **incomplete histories**. Repeated use of old notes can perpetuate inaccuracies, fail to reflect the patient's current status, and overlook important changes in their condition.
    - To avoid this pitfall, clinicians should always **customize and update notes** for each encounter, ensuring that the patient's current concerns, symptoms, and history are accurately recorded. Consistently reviewing and revising the history improves the accuracy of the medical record and enhances clinical decision-making .

References

- Croskerry, P. "Diagnostic Failure: A Cognitive and Affective Approach." *BMJ Quality & Safety*, 2018.
- Hoffman, K., et al. "Implicit Bias in Healthcare Professionals: A Systematic Review." *BMC Medical Ethics*, 2020.
- Roter, D. L., et al. "Patient Participation in the Patient-Provider Interaction: The Effects of Patient Question Asking on the Quality of Interaction, Satisfaction and Compliance." *Medical Care*, 2019.
- Beckman, H. B., et al. "The Doctor-Patient Relationship and Malpractice: Lessons from Plaintiff Depositions." *Archives of Internal Medicine*, 2018.
- Booth, N., et al. "Can We Really Measure Implicit Bias? Understanding the Pros and Cons of Implicit Association Tests in Healthcare." *Journal of Clinical Psychology*, 2020.
- Street, R. L., et al. "The Impact of Computer Use on Physician-Patient Communication in the Exam Room." *Journal of the American Medical Informatics Association*, 2017.
- Shachak, A., et al. "Impact of Electronic Medical Records on Physician-Patient Communication: A Systematic Review." *Journal of the American Medical Informatics Association*, 2019.
- Frankel, R. M., et al. "Medical Visit Time and Physician-Patient Communication: A Critical Review." *Journal of General Internal Medicine*, 2021.
- Gossman, W., et al. "Use of the EMR: Balancing Physician Efficiency and Patient Care." *Journal of Health Informatics*, 2020.
- Sinsky, C., et al. "Restoring Primary Care: What Physicians Can Do to Reconnect with Patients and Revitalize Practice." *Journal of General Internal Medicine*, 2021.

Chapter 7: History Taking in Acute Situations and Telemedicine

In acute and emergency settings, clinicians must adapt their history-taking techniques to gather essential information quickly and efficiently. This focused approach helps prioritize life-saving interventions while obtaining enough information to guide diagnosis and treatment.

A. Focused History in Critical Care

1. **Rapid History Taking in Trauma and Medical Emergencies**:
    - In **trauma** and **medical emergencies**, history taking must be concise, focusing on information that can guide immediate care. Time-sensitive conditions like **cardiac arrest**, **trauma**, or **sepsis** require a rapid assessment to prioritize life-saving interventions.
    - The **primary survey** (ABCDE: **Airway, Breathing, Circulation, Disability, Exposure**) addresses immediate life threats, while history taking is performed concurrently or immediately after stabilization. In trauma cases, the **mechanism of injury** can provide crucial clues about potential internal damage, and asking about the use of **seat belts**, **helmets**, or the **height of a fall** can guide decision-making about imaging and surgery.
    - For medical emergencies such as **myocardial infarction** or **stroke**, quick, focused questions about the **onset** of symptoms, previous episodes, and any use of medications (e.g., anticoagulants or antiplatelets) are critical for guiding treatment decisions such as **thrombolysis** or **percutaneous coronary intervention (PCI)**.
2. **Prioritizing the Most Critical Information (AMPLE: Allergies, Medications, Past Medical History, Last Meal, Events Leading Up)**:
    - The **AMPLE** mnemonic is a well-established approach for gathering crucial information quickly in emergencies:
        - **A**: **Allergies** – Identifying any known allergies, particularly to **medications**, **latex**, or **contrast agents**, is essential before administering emergency medications or performing procedures.
        - **M**: **Medications** – Asking about current **medications** helps avoid drug interactions and identifies potential overdose situations. **Anticoagulants**, for instance, are critical to know in trauma or head injury cases due to the risk of **bleeding**.
        - **P**: **Past Medical History** – This includes **chronic conditions** such as diabetes, heart disease, and asthma, which may affect emergency management decisions (e.g., adjusting insulin in diabetic ketoacidosis or managing asthma exacerbations).
        - **L**: **Last Meal** – Knowing the patient's **last oral intake** is important, particularly if surgery or sedation is anticipated, to reduce the risk of aspiration.
        - **E**: **Events Leading Up** – Clarifying the sequence of events before the emergency, such as the onset of pain, trauma mechanism, or preceding

symptoms, can provide essential diagnostic clues. For example, understanding whether chest pain began at rest or with exertion can guide the differential diagnosis between **stable angina**, **unstable angina**, or **myocardial infarction**.
3. Using **AMPLE** helps the clinician gather targeted, life-saving information without overwhelming the patient with unnecessary questions in high-stress situations. Studies show that following structured formats like AMPLE improves diagnostic accuracy and reduces errors in emergency settings.

B. Telephone and Remote History Taking

1. **Adapting History-Taking Techniques for Telemedicine**:
   - With the expansion of **telemedicine** during the COVID-19 pandemic, history-taking skills have been adapted to suit **virtual consultations**. In the absence of a physical exam, obtaining a thorough and detailed history is even more critical.
   - Clinicians must rely on the patient's description of symptoms and use **open-ended questions** to gather as much information as possible. For example, when assessing **chest pain** via telemedicine, it is crucial to ask detailed questions about the **location**, **quality**, and **radiation** of the pain to distinguish between musculoskeletal causes and more serious conditions like angina or pulmonary embolism.
   - Visual cues, such as observing **respiratory effort**, **facial expression**, or the **presence of rash**, can still be valuable during telemedicine encounters. Asking the patient to **show** certain body parts or perform self-examinations (e.g., taking their own pulse or checking for swelling) can provide useful additional data.
   - **Telemedicine platforms** should be used to integrate **secure messaging**, **video**, and **remote monitoring tools** to supplement history taking and enhance diagnosis. Remote monitoring devices, such as **blood pressure cuffs**, **pulse oximeters**, and **glucometers**, can provide real-time data to clinicians, further improving the accuracy of remote consultations.

2. **Ensuring Thoroughness in the Absence of Physical Examination**:
   - One of the challenges of telemedicine is ensuring that the history is thorough enough to compensate for the lack of a **physical examination**. Clinicians must ask more detailed questions about symptoms that would typically be assessed through physical signs. For instance, in evaluating **shortness of breath**, the physician might ask the patient to describe how far they can walk before becoming short of breath, and whether the symptoms worsen when lying flat (to assess for **orthopnea**).
   - Using validated **clinical decision tools** can help in remote settings. For example, the **Wells Criteria** for pulmonary embolism can guide the need for further testing based on the patient's history of symptoms like **leg swelling**, **recent immobilization**, or **hemoptysis**.

- A systematic approach to history taking in telemedicine, such as using checklists or following a symptom-based algorithm, ensures that critical information is not missed. Studies indicate that structured history-taking protocols in telemedicine improve diagnostic accuracy and patient satisfaction .
3. Additionally, it's important to **set patient expectations** during remote consultations. Explain the limitations of virtual visits and ensure that patients know when they need to seek in-person care. For example, if a patient presents with **chest pain**, it may be necessary to advise them to visit an emergency department for further evaluation.

References

1. Moulton, C., et al. "Emergency Medical History Taking: A Critical Review." *Journal of Emergency Medicine*, 2020.
2. Croskerry, P. "The Importance of Thinking Clearly and Quickly: Diagnostic Decision-Making in the Emergency Department." *BMJ Quality & Safety*, 2018.
3. Carley, S., et al. "Trauma Emergencies: Gathering Essential Information Rapidly." *Annals of Emergency Medicine*, 2019.
4. Sinsky, C., et al. "The Expansion of Telemedicine and Its Impact on Clinical History Taking: A Review of Current Practices." *Journal of Telemedicine and Telecare*, 2021.
5. Greenhalgh, T., et al. "Covid-19: A Remote Assessment in Primary Care." *BMJ*, 2020.
6. Shachak, A., et al. "Impact of Telemedicine on Clinical Communication: Opportunities and Challenges." *Journal of Telemedicine and eHealth*, 2020.
7. Kessler, C. S., et al. "History Taking in the Emergency Department: Defining the Role of AMPLE." *Journal of Emergency Nursing*, 2018.
8. Schwamm, L. H., et al. "Recommendations for the Implementation of Telemedicine within Stroke Systems of Care." *Stroke*, 2020.
9. White, S., et al. "History Taking in Critical Care Settings: The Role of Focused Interviews in Trauma Cases." *Trauma Surgery & Acute Care Open*, 2020.

Chapter 8: Integrating History Taking with Physical Examination

A. **Putting Information Together**

1. **How to Connect History with Physical Findings**:
    - The **integration of history taking with physical examination** is essential in diagnosing and managing patient care. A comprehensive history provides the framework for understanding the patient's symptoms, and the physical exam allows for the **validation or refinement** of hypotheses generated during the interview. The goal is to create a **cohesive narrative** that links patient-reported symptoms with objective findings.
    - For example, a patient presenting with **chest pain** described as pressure-like and radiating to the left arm (classic for angina) may have physical exam findings such as **elevated jugular venous pressure (JVP)** and **bibasilar crackles**, suggesting **heart failure** secondary to ischemia. In this case, the history of **chest pain** aligns with physical signs of **heart failure**, guiding the clinician toward a diagnosis of **acute coronary syndrome** or **acute decompensated heart failure**.
    - Studies show that physicians who effectively integrate history and physical examination findings make more accurate diagnoses compared to those who focus on one aspect alone. The combination of subjective and objective information leads to a **higher diagnostic yield**, emphasizing the importance of synthesis in clinical practice.
2. **Recognizing Patterns in Common Diseases**:
    - Certain patterns in **history** and **physical findings** are associated with common diseases. By recognizing these patterns, clinicians can more quickly identify potential diagnoses and avoid unnecessary testing.
        - For example, a patient with a history of **morning joint stiffness** lasting more than 30 minutes, combined with physical exam findings of **symmetric joint swelling**, may have **rheumatoid arthritis**.
        - A patient with a **cough** and **fever**, combined with **crackles** or **dullness to percussion** on lung exam, suggests **pneumonia**.
    - By recognizing patterns like these, clinicians can use history and physical examination findings to streamline the diagnostic process, reduce the need for extensive testing, and begin treatment more rapidly. Studies suggest that early recognition of clinical patterns improves patient outcomes by facilitating timely interventions.
3. **Using History to Guide the Physical Exam Focus**:
    - The **history** should guide the clinician in focusing the **physical examination** on relevant systems and areas of concern. This ensures that the physical exam is both **efficient and targeted**, reducing unnecessary steps and focusing on key diagnostic clues.
    - For instance, a patient with a history of **dyspnea on exertion** and **orthopnea** should prompt a physical exam that emphasizes **cardiovascular and**

pulmonary assessments, including inspection for **jugular venous distension**, palpation for the **point of maximal impulse (PMI)**, auscultation for **S3 or S4 heart sounds**, and evaluation for **rales or wheezes** in the lungs.
- In patients with **abdominal pain**, the history may direct the clinician to focus on **abdominal examination**, including palpation for tenderness, masses, **rebound tenderness**, and **Murphy's sign**, depending on the location and nature of the pain. A focused physical exam, based on the history, is more likely to reveal the critical findings needed for diagnosis.

B. Differential Diagnosis Development

1. **Structuring a Differential Diagnosis Based on History**:
   - A thorough **history** provides the foundation for developing a **differential diagnosis**. Clinicians must use the information gathered to create a list of potential diagnoses, ranked by likelihood, while considering **common diseases** first and remaining alert to **life-threatening conditions**.
   - The **mnemonic VINDICATE** can be helpful in organizing differential diagnoses:
     - **V**: **Vascular** (e.g., stroke, myocardial infarction)
     - **I**: **Infectious** (e.g., pneumonia, meningitis)
     - **N**: **Neoplastic** (e.g., lung cancer, colon cancer)
     - **D**: **Degenerative** (e.g., osteoarthritis)
     - **I**: **Inflammatory**/Autoimmune (e.g., lupus, rheumatoid arthritis)
     - **C**: **Congenital** (e.g., congenital heart disease)
     - **A**: **Allergic**/Anaphylactic (e.g., asthma, anaphylaxis)
     - **T**: **Traumatic** (e.g., fractures, head injury)
     - **E**: **Endocrine/Metabolic** (e.g., diabetes, hypothyroidism)
   - For example, a patient presenting with **fever**, **pleuritic chest pain**, and **productive cough** might have a differential diagnosis that includes **bacterial pneumonia, viral pneumonia, pulmonary embolism**, and **lung cancer**. The history would guide the clinician in prioritizing bacterial pneumonia if the patient has associated **chills**, **colored sputum**, and a history of recent illness.
2. **Determining the Next Steps in Diagnostic Work-Up**:
   - Once a differential diagnosis is established, the clinician must determine the most appropriate **next steps** in the diagnostic work-up. The choice of tests should be guided by the **most likely diagnoses** and the need to **rule out life-threatening conditions**.
   - For instance, in a patient with **chest pain** and concern for **acute coronary syndrome**, the next steps would include obtaining an **electrocardiogram (ECG)**, measuring **troponin levels**, and possibly performing **cardiac catheterization** if indicated. A thorough history and well-conducted physical examination direct these decisions and prevent unnecessary or redundant testing.

- Similarly, in a patient with **abdominal pain** and concern for **appendicitis**, the work-up might include **ultrasound** or **CT imaging**, guided by findings such as **McBurney's point tenderness** on physical examination.
- Studies have shown that using history to guide the diagnostic work-up can reduce the use of unnecessary tests and imaging, leading to more cost-effective care without compromising diagnostic accuracy .

3. Additionally, when determining the next steps, it's essential to consider **patient-specific factors** such as age, comorbidities, and risk factors, which may influence the choice of diagnostic tests. For example, elderly patients with **vague abdominal pain** are more likely to have serious conditions like **mesenteric ischemia**, prompting earlier imaging than in younger patients with similar symptoms.

References

- McGee, S. "Evidence-Based Physical Diagnosis." 4th ed., Elsevier, 2017.
- Bickley, L. S. "Bates' Guide to Physical Examination and History Taking." 13th ed., Wolters Kluwer, 2021.
- Norman, G., et al. "Diagnostic Reasoning and the Clinical Examination." *Journal of the American Medical Association*, 2020.
- Groopman, J. E. "How Doctors Think." Houghton Mifflin, 2018.
- Croskerry, P. "The Importance of Cognitive Strategies in Diagnosis." *BMJ Quality & Safety*, 2021.
- Murtagh, J. "General Practice: History and Clinical Examination." 6th ed., McGraw-Hill, 2020.
- Durning, S. J., et al. "The Importance of Clinical Reasoning in Diagnostic Excellence." *New England Journal of Medicine*, 2021.
- Schwamm, L. H., et al. "Improving Diagnostic Accuracy by Synthesizing History and Physical Examination." *Annals of Internal Medicine*, 2019.

Chapter 9: Examples of History Taking of Common Conditions at Wynn Medical Center

1. Diabetes Mellitus (Type 2)

Case Example:
A 50-year-old Chinese male presents for a routine check-up and reports **increased thirst** and **frequent urination** over the last three months.

History Focus:

- **Onset**: Ask when the symptoms began.
- **Polyuria/Polydipsia**: Inquire about **frequency of urination**, **nocturia**, and whether **increased fluid intake** is related to thirst.
- **Weight changes**: Ask about **recent weight loss or gain**.
- **Fatigue**: Inquire about persistent **fatigue** or **blurred vision**.
- **Family history**: Ask about a family history of **diabetes** or related conditions like **hypertension** or **heart disease**.
- **Complications**: Ask about any signs of **peripheral neuropathy** (e.g., numbness, tingling), **visual changes**, or **non-healing wounds**.
- **Medications**: Inquire about current treatment, including **oral hypoglycemic agents** or **insulin**, and adherence to these medications.

Clinical Significance:
The symptoms of **polydipsia**, **polyuria**, and **unexplained weight loss** are classic for **new-onset or poorly controlled diabetes mellitus**. A targeted history can guide the next steps, including obtaining an **HbA1c** or **fasting glucose** to confirm the diagnosis or assess control.

---

2. Hyperlipidemia

Case Example:
A 45-year-old Vietnamese woman presents for routine health maintenance and reports no specific symptoms but is concerned about her **family history of heart disease**.

History Focus:

- **Risk factors**: Ask about **smoking, alcohol intake, diet, physical activity**, and family history of **coronary artery disease (CAD)**, especially premature CAD.
- **Past lipid levels**: Inquire about previous **cholesterol measurements**, whether they've been high, and if the patient is on **lipid-lowering medications**.
- **Symptoms of CAD**: Ask about **chest pain, shortness of breath**, or **leg pain on exertion** (claudication).
- **Diet and exercise**: Inquire about the patient's typical diet and level of **physical activity**.

Clinical Significance:
Even in the absence of symptoms, hyperlipidemia is a significant risk factor for **atherosclerotic cardiovascular disease**. This history will guide whether to initiate or adjust **statin therapy** and recommend lifestyle modifications.

---

3. Wrist Pain

Case Example:
A 35-year-old Korean administrative assistant presents with **right wrist pain** that has been worsening over the past month, especially while typing.

History Focus:

- **Onset**: Ask about when the pain started and any precipitating events.
- **Location**: Focus on the **specific area of pain** in the wrist (e.g., dorsal vs. palmar surface).
- **Character**: Inquire if the pain is **sharp, dull, or throbbing**.
- **Aggravating/relieving factors**: Ask about activities that make the pain worse (e.g., typing, gripping objects) and what relieves it (e.g., rest, ice).
- **Numbness/tingling**: Ask if there is **numbness** or **tingling** in the fingers, especially in the **thumb**, **index**, or **middle fingers**, which may suggest **carpal tunnel syndrome**.
- **Injury history**: Ask about any history of **trauma** or repetitive **strain**.

Clinical Significance:
The patient's occupation and symptoms suggest **repetitive strain injury** or **carpal tunnel syndrome**. A targeted physical exam, including **Tinel's sign** and **Phalen's maneuver**, can help confirm the diagnosis.

---

4. Urinary Tract Infection (UTI)

Case Example:
A 30-year-old African female presents with **dysuria, increased urinary frequency**, and **suprapubic discomfort** for three days.

History Focus:

- **Onset**: Ask when the symptoms began.
- **Urinary symptoms**: Inquire about the **frequency**, **urgency**, and whether urination is painful.
- **Associated symptoms**: Ask about **hematuria, fever, flank pain**, or **nausea/vomiting** to rule out **pyelonephritis**.

- **Sexual history**: Inquire about recent sexual activity, as sexually transmitted infections can present similarly.
- **Previous UTIs**: Ask about any prior UTIs and the effectiveness of past treatments.

Clinical Significance:
This presentation is classic for **acute cystitis**. The absence of fever and flank pain lowers suspicion for more complicated infections like **pyelonephritis**.

---

5. Psoriasis

Case Example:
A 40-year-old Vietnamese male presents with **itchy, red, scaly patches** on his scalp, elbows, and knees that have worsened over the past six months.

History Focus:

- **Onset**: When did the lesions first appear, and how have they progressed?
- **Location**: Focus on areas commonly affected by **psoriasis** (scalp, elbows, knees).
- **Character**: Ask about the **itchiness**, **pain**, or **scaliness** of the lesions.
- **Associated symptoms**: Inquire about **nail changes** (pitting, onycholysis) or **joint pain** to evaluate for **psoriatic arthritis**.
- **Family history**: Ask if other family members have psoriasis or autoimmune diseases.

Clinical Significance:
The history of **chronic, scaly plaques** in typical locations suggests **psoriasis**. A physical exam and possible **biopsy** can confirm the diagnosis, guiding treatment with **topical corticosteroids** or **systemic agents**.

---

6. Osteoarthritis

Case Example:
A 62-year-old Thai woman presents with **chronic knee pain** that worsens throughout the day and after prolonged activity.

History Focus:

- **Onset**: Ask how long the pain has been present and if there was any **injury** to the knee.
- **Character**: Inquire if the pain is **deep, aching**, and **worse with activity**.
- **Morning stiffness**: Ask if the stiffness lasts <30 minutes in the morning.
- **Functional limitations**: Inquire about difficulty with **walking**, **climbing stairs**, or **sitting down**.
- **Past injuries**: Ask about any **previous joint injuries** or surgeries.

Clinical Significance:
The history of **activity-related joint pain** and **morning stiffness** suggests **osteoarthritis**. This will prompt imaging (e.g., **X-ray**) to assess for joint space narrowing and guide treatment with **physical therapy**, **NSAIDs**, or **joint injections**.

---

7. Chest Pain

Case Example:
A 55-year-old male presents with **chest pain** that occurs with exertion and resolves with rest. He has a history of **hypertension** and **smoking**.

History Focus:

- **Onset**: Ask when the pain began and if it was sudden or gradual.
- **Quality**: Ask how the pain feels (e.g., **pressure-like**, **sharp**, **burning**).
- **Radiation**: Inquire if the pain radiates to the **jaw**, **neck**, or **arms**.
- **Associated symptoms**: Ask about **shortness of breath**, **diaphoresis**, **nausea**, or **dizziness**.
- **Risk factors**: Ask about risk factors for coronary artery disease, including **hypertension**, **diabetes**, **hyperlipidemia**, and a history of **smoking**.

Clinical Significance:
The classic presentation of **exertional chest pain** relieved by rest suggests **stable angina**. Immediate evaluation with an **ECG** and possibly **stress testing** or **cardiac catheterization** is warranted.

---

8. Upper Respiratory Infection (URI)

Case Example:
A 25-year-old female presents with **nasal congestion**, **sore throat**, and **cough** for five days.

History Focus:

- **Onset**: When did the symptoms start, and how have they progressed?
- **Fever**: Ask if the patient has had a fever.
- **Sore throat**: Inquire about **pain with swallowing** or **hoarseness**.
- **Cough**: Ask about the nature of the cough (dry vs. productive) and if there is **colored sputum**.
- **Ear pain or sinus pressure**: Ask about **ear pain**, **headache**, or **facial pain**, which could indicate sinusitis or otitis media.

Clinical Significance:
The patient's symptoms suggest a **viral URI**, and treatment is likely **supportive**, including hydration and over-the-counter remedies. Any **fever**, **persistent symptoms**, or signs of bacterial infection might require further evaluation.

---

9. Abdominal Pain

Case Example:
A 40-year-old male presents with **right upper quadrant pain** after eating fatty meals, which has been occurring for the past two weeks.

History Focus:

- **Onset**: Ask how long the pain has been present and whether it is related to meals.
- **Location**: Focus on the **right upper quadrant** and if the pain radiates to the **back** or **shoulder**.
- **Character**: Inquire if the pain is **sharp, cramping, or dull**.
- **Aggravating/relieving factors**: Ask if the pain worsens after eating fatty foods and if it improves with rest.
- **Associated symptoms**: Inquire about **nausea**, **vomiting**, **fever**, or **jaundice**.

Clinical Significance:
The patient's history suggests **biliary colic**, likely due to **cholelithiasis** or **cholecystitis**. Further evaluation with **abdominal ultrasound** is indicated.

---

10. Cervical Radiculopathy

Case Example:
A 45-year-old male presents with **neck pain** and **tingling** in his right arm, worsened by turning his head.

History Focus:

- **Onset**: Ask when the symptoms began and if there was any trauma.
- **Pain description**: Inquire if the pain is **sharp, burning, or aching**.
- **Radiation**: Ask about radiation of pain into the **shoulder**, **arm**, or **fingers**.
- **Numbness/weakness**: Ask about **numbness**, **tingling**, or **muscle weakness** in the arm.
- **Aggravating/relieving factors**: Ask if the pain worsens with certain neck positions and improves with rest.

Clinical Significance:
The history is suggestive of **cervical radiculopathy**. A focused physical exam and **MRI** of the cervical spine can help confirm the diagnosis and guide treatment with **physical therapy**, **pain management**, or possible **surgical intervention**.

---

11. Low Back Pain

Case Example:
A 50-year-old Chinese female presents with **low back pain** that began two weeks ago after lifting a heavy object.

History Focus:

- **Onset**: Ask if the pain started suddenly or gradually.
- **Character**: Inquire if the pain is **dull**, **sharp**, or **shooting**.
- **Radiation**: Ask if the pain radiates down the legs, which could indicate **sciatica**.
- **Aggravating/relieving factors**: Ask what worsens the pain (e.g., bending, standing) and what relieves it (e.g., lying down).
- **Red flags**: Inquire about **bowel or bladder incontinence**, **numbness in the groin area**, **fever**, or **weight loss**, which could suggest more serious conditions like **cauda equina syndrome** or **malignancy**.

Clinical Significance:
The history suggests **mechanical low back pain** due to strain. However, any **red flags** would prompt urgent imaging and further evaluation.

References:

- Bickley, L. S. *Bates' Guide to Physical Examination and History Taking.* 13th ed., Wolters Kluwer, 2021.
- McGee, S. *Evidence-Based Physical Diagnosis.* 4th ed., Elsevier, 2017.
- Dains, J. E., et al. *Advanced Health Assessment and Clinical Diagnosis in Primary Care.* 6th ed., Elsevier, 2020.

Part 2: The Physical Exam

Chapter 10: Why is the physical exam important?

The physical examination is a cornerstone of clinical practice, particularly for internal medicine medical students, residents, advanced pharmacist practitioner residents, and NP residents.

While advances in diagnostic imaging and laboratory testing have transformed medical diagnostics, the physical exam remains an essential skill that provides immediate, cost-effective, and valuable information about a patient's health. Studies have shown that a well-performed physical examination can identify diagnostic clues that may not be evident through imaging or laboratory results alone .

Moreover, the physical examination fosters the doctor-patient relationship. A study by Verghese et al. emphasized that the act of physical examination contributes to building trust between physicians and patients, which is vital for patient compliance and outcomes . In internal medicine, residents must develop a refined ability to gather clinical information through history and physical examination, as this influences the initial diagnostic hypotheses and subsequent decisions regarding testing and treatment .

In the context of internal medicine and outpatient family practice, physical exams are particularly important for conditions such as heart failure, pneumonia, liver disease, and autoimmune disorders, where clinical signs may lead to an early diagnosis and proper management. Mastering these skills early in residency provides a foundation for developing clinical intuition and improving diagnostic accuracy.

A. Role of Physical Examination in Clinical Decision-Making

The physical exam is not only a diagnostic tool but also plays a pivotal role in decision-making throughout the patient's care. Research suggests that up to 20-25% of diagnoses in internal medicine are based primarily on history and physical examination . A skilled physical examination can direct the clinician toward or away from certain diagnoses, reducing unnecessary tests and minimizing healthcare costs.

For example, assessing jugular venous pressure (JVP) and auscultating for heart murmurs can lead to earlier recognition of heart failure, often before lab results become available . Similarly, examining for hepatosplenomegaly or ascites can provide immediate insight into liver disease. The efficiency and effectiveness of these examinations are critical in emergency and resource-limited settings, where advanced diagnostic tools may not be readily accessible .

By developing competence in physical examination, residents are empowered to make informed decisions at the bedside, potentially initiating treatment before confirmatory testing. This immediacy can be lifesaving in acute situations and is especially relevant for complex cases in internal medicine.

B. How to Use This Book

This book is structured to guide internal medicine students/residents, APP residents, and NP residents through a systematic approach to physical examination, beginning with general principles and progressing through system-specific chapters. Each chapter follows a consistent format:

1. Introduction: Brief overview of the anatomy and physiology relevant to the system being examined.
2. Examination Techniques: Step-by-step instructions for conducting the exam, emphasizing key findings.
3. Common Findings: Descriptions of normal and abnormal findings, with clinical correlations.
4. Case Studies: Real-life clinical scenarios to highlight the importance of the exam findings and how they inform diagnosis and management.

The book also integrates evidence-based guidelines to ensure that residents are learning not only traditional techniques but also those validated by recent research.

C. Practical Tips for Integrating Physical Exam Skills into Daily Practice

For internal medicine residents, balancing the demands of patient care with continuous skill development can be challenging. To aid in this process, this book provides practical tips for integrating physical exam techniques into daily routines:

1. Perform focused exams on every patient: While full head-to-toe examinations may not be necessary for every visit, practicing focused exams based on patient complaints reinforces skills without overwhelming the resident.
2. Use the exam to guide further testing: Incorporating exam findings to justify lab orders or imaging can sharpen clinical reasoning. For instance, in a patient with suspected pneumonia, consolidating lung findings with imaging results helps reinforce clinical skills.
3. Incorporate POCUS (point-of-care ultrasound): Whenever possible, residents should use bedside ultrasound to enhance their physical exam skills, especially for evaluating the heart, lungs, and abdomen.

These small, daily efforts can significantly improve diagnostic accuracy over time and help the resident internalize key examination techniques.

D. Common Pitfalls and How to Avoid Them

Even experienced physicians can make errors during physical exams, which can lead to misdiagnosis. Common pitfalls include:

1. Over-reliance on technology: Modern medicine often overemphasizes diagnostic imaging and lab tests, which can lead to overlooking crucial physical exam findings. Studies have shown that physical examination skills deteriorate when not practiced regularly . This book emphasizes the importance of integrating physical exam skills with technology, rather than substituting one for the other.

2. Rushed exams: Time pressure during rounds or clinic visits may lead to incomplete or superficial exams. This can be mitigated by focusing on efficiency without sacrificing thoroughness. For example, prioritizing key systems based on the presenting symptoms can streamline the exam without missing essential findings.
3. Lack of consistency: Inconsistent examination techniques can lead to variability in findings. This book encourages a systematic approach to ensure that exams are performed in the same way every time. Developing a consistent routine will help reduce missed findings and improve diagnostic reliability.

By identifying these common pitfalls, residents can take proactive steps to improve their clinical examination skills, ensuring they become adept at using the physical exam to its full potential.

References

- Mangione, S. "Physical Diagnosis Secrets." 4th ed., Elsevier, 2018.
- McGee, S. "Evidence-Based Physical Diagnosis." 4th ed., Elsevier, 2017.
- Verghese, A. "The Importance of the Physical Examination in Clinical Medicine." BMJ, 2011.
- Reilly, B. M. "Physical Examination in the Care of Medical Inpatients: An Observational Study." Lancet, 2003.
- Peterson, M. C. "Contributions of the History, Physical Examination, and Laboratory Investigation in Making Medical Diagnoses." Western Journal of Medicine, 1992.
- Joffe, M. P., et al. "Physical Examination Skills: Closing the Gap Between Medical School and Residency." Academic Medicine, 2015.
- Franco-Sadud, R., et al. "Point-of-Care Ultrasound: Applications in Critical Care." Cleveland Clinic Journal of Medicine, 2019.
- Elder, A., Japp, A. "How Confident Are Doctors in Using Their Stethoscope? A Cross-Sectional Study." BMJ Open, 2016.

Chapter 11: General Principles of the Physical Examination

A. How to Prepare the Patient and the Environment for the Exam

Before performing a physical examination, it is essential to ensure that both the patient and the environment are adequately prepared. This preparation not only makes the examination more efficient but also enhances patient comfort and the quality of the findings.

1. Setting the Environment:
   The examination room should be quiet, well-lit, and appropriately equipped with all necessary tools (stethoscope, otoscope, ophthalmoscope, reflex hammer, etc.). A clean, organized workspace minimizes distractions and enhances focus on the patient. Privacy should be ensured by closing doors or using curtains, and the patient should be offered a gown to promote comfort and dignity during the exam . Adjust the temperature of the room to ensure it's comfortable, as patients may feel cold during an exam if undressed.
2. Positioning the Patient:
   Patients should be positioned in a way that allows for easy access to the areas being examined. For instance, in a cardiovascular or respiratory exam, the patient should be seated at a 45-degree angle to allow for optimal examination of the jugular venous pressure and breath sounds. Ensuring that the patient is comfortable and appropriately draped is key to reducing anxiety and enhancing cooperation during the exam .

B. Communication Skills: Explaining the Exam to the Patient

Effective communication is integral to establishing trust and ensuring that the patient understands the purpose of the physical examination. This is particularly important for sensitive exams or when examining children and elderly patients.

1. Explain the Process:
   Prior to the exam, explain each step to the patient in simple, understandable terms. For example, say, "I am going to listen to your lungs to check how well you are breathing." This not only reduces anxiety but also fosters collaboration and encourages patients to share relevant information about their symptoms . Research shows that patients are more likely to disclose important details when they feel informed and involved in the process .
2. Seek Consent:
   Always ask for consent before proceeding with any physical contact. This is particularly important during intimate or invasive parts of the exam. Using phrases such as, "Is it okay if I check your abdomen now?" ensures that the patient feels respected and retains a sense of control throughout the process . The practice of gaining consent not only complies with ethical standards but also fosters a positive doctor-patient relationship.
3. Reassure the Patient:
   Reassurance can be verbal ("This might feel a little cold, but it won't hurt") or non-verbal

(maintaining eye contact, using a calm tone of voice). This can make a big difference, especially with pediatric or anxious patients. A study published in *Patient Education and Counseling* highlighted that clear communication and reassurance significantly reduce patient discomfort and anxiety during physical exams .

C. Systematic Approach to the Physical Exam

1. Head-to-Toe vs. Focused Exam Approaches:
   A head-to-toe exam is typically used in routine physicals or when patients present with vague or non-specific symptoms. This systematic approach ensures that no body system is overlooked and provides a comprehensive view of the patient's health status. It is particularly useful for initial evaluations or in the inpatient setting, where a complete understanding of the patient's overall condition is needed .
   In contrast, a focused exam is directed at the primary complaint. For instance, if a patient presents with chest pain, the examination will focus on the cardiovascular and respiratory systems. This approach saves time and helps to narrow down differential diagnoses. The choice between these approaches depends on the clinical context.
2. Documentation and Reporting of Physical Findings:
   Accurate documentation of physical exam findings is critical in medical practice. This includes describing what was examined, how it was done, and the results. It is important to use precise, standardized terminology. For instance, describing heart sounds as "normal S1 and S2 without murmurs, rubs, or gallops" communicates clear, detailed information. Moreover, any abnormal findings should be described in terms of their location, size, shape, and quality (e.g., "2 cm, round, non-tender nodule on the thyroid gland"). Documentation not only serves as a legal record but also helps to track changes over time and communicates findings to other healthcare professionals involved in the patient's care .
3. Combining Clinical Reasoning with the Physical Exam:
   The physical exam is not a standalone procedure but rather part of a larger clinical reasoning process. Each finding should be interpreted in the context of the patient's history and current symptoms. For example, discovering lower extremity edema in a patient with shortness of breath might point to heart failure, whereas the same finding in a patient with liver disease may suggest cirrhosis. Clinical reasoning involves constantly integrating new information to refine diagnostic hypotheses and guide further testing or treatment .

D. Infection Control and Hygiene

1. Hand Hygiene and Proper Use of PPE During Exams:
   Hand hygiene is the single most effective way to prevent the spread of infections in healthcare settings. Before and after each patient encounter, clinicians must wash their

hands with soap and water or use an alcohol-based hand sanitizer, following established guidelines from the Centers for Disease Control and Prevention (CDC). Proper hand hygiene prevents the transmission of pathogens between patients and from the clinician to the patient .

2. Personal Protective Equipment (PPE):

In certain situations, PPE such as gloves, masks, or gowns may be required to protect both the patient and the healthcare provider from infection. For example, gloves should be worn during invasive procedures or when contact with bodily fluids is anticipated. Additionally, wearing masks may be necessary in cases where respiratory infections are suspected, such as during flu season or in patients with tuberculosis . Infection control practices became especially crucial during the COVID-19 pandemic, where guidelines evolved to protect both patients and healthcare providers from airborne and droplet transmission .

Adhering to these hygiene protocols not only ensures the safety of both the patient and healthcare provider but also reassures patients, many of whom are increasingly aware of infection control issues due to heightened media attention during global health crises .

References

- Smith, L. A., et al. "Environmental Factors in the Examination Room and Their Impact on Patient Comfort." *Journal of General Internal Medicine*, 2017.
- Verghese, A., et al. "The Importance of Bedside Medicine in Clinical Diagnosis." *New England Journal of Medicine*, 2011.
- Kelley, M. A., et al. "Effective Communication During Patient Examinations: Reducing Anxiety and Improving Outcomes." *Patient Education and Counseling*, 2016.
- Epstein, R. M., & Street, R. L. "Patient-Centered Communication in Health Care." *American Psychological Association*, 2007.
- Bickley, L. S., & Szilagyi, P. G. "Bates' Guide to Physical Examination and History Taking." 13th ed., Wolters Kluwer, 2021.
- World Health Organization. "Infection Prevention and Control: Hand Hygiene." *WHO*, 2020.
- Siegel, J. D., et al. "Guideline for Isolation Precautions: Preventing Transmission of Infectious Agents in Healthcare Settings." *Centers for Disease Control and Prevention*, 2019.

Chapter 12. Vital Signs and General Appearance

A. Blood Pressure Measurement Techniques

Blood pressure (BP) measurement is a fundamental part of the physical exam and is crucial in detecting hypertension, hypotension, and cardiovascular risk. Accurate BP measurement relies on proper technique, and studies have shown that incorrect procedures can lead to inaccurate readings, which may result in misdiagnosis and inappropriate management of conditions like hypertension .

1. **Manual vs. Automated BP Measurement:**
    - Manual BP measurement using a sphygmomanometer and stethoscope remains the gold standard, especially in clinical settings where precision is necessary. The Korotkoff sounds are used to determine systolic and diastolic pressures, and proper technique involves inflating the cuff to about 20-30 mmHg above the point where the radial pulse disappears .
    - Automated BP monitors are increasingly used for convenience and standardization in busy clinical settings, especially for patients who need frequent monitoring. However, their accuracy can be affected by factors such as improper cuff size or patient movement .
2. **Proper Technique for Accurate BP Measurement:**
    - Positioning the patient: The patient should be seated comfortably with their back supported and feet flat on the floor. The arm should be supported at heart level, and the cuff should be wrapped around the upper arm, ensuring it is neither too tight nor too loose. A cuff that is too small can lead to falsely elevated readings, while a cuff that is too large can produce falsely low readings .
    - Conditions before measurement: The patient should rest for at least 5 minutes before the measurement, avoiding talking or movement. If BP is measured after physical activity, eating, or smoking, the results may not accurately reflect the patient's baseline blood pressure .
    - Multiple readings: In clinical practice, it is recommended to take at least two readings, 1-2 minutes apart, and average them. In cases of significant discrepancies, additional measurements should be taken .

B. Pulse, Respiratory Rate, Temperature, and Oxygen Saturation Interpretation

1. **Pulse:**
    - The pulse rate is typically measured at the radial artery and is an important indicator of cardiovascular health. The normal range for adults is between 60-100 beats per minute (bpm), though athletes may have lower resting heart rates . Bradycardia (pulse < 60 bpm) can suggest underlying heart block or medication effects (e.g., beta-blockers), while tachycardia (pulse > 100 bpm) may indicate fever, dehydration, or systemic issues such as sepsis or hyperthyroidism .

- Pulse quality (e.g., strong, weak, thready, or bounding) can provide insight into cardiac output or peripheral vascular resistance. A bounding pulse may suggest hyperthyroidism, aortic insufficiency, or fever, while a weak, thready pulse can be seen in shock or heart failure.

2. **Respiratory Rate (RR):**
    - The normal respiratory rate for adults is 12-20 breaths per minute. Tachypnea (RR > 20) may indicate respiratory distress, metabolic acidosis, or other pulmonary pathology, whereas bradypnea (RR < 12) could suggest central nervous system depression or metabolic alkalosis.
    - Observing the pattern and depth of breathing is also essential. For example, Kussmaul breathing (deep, labored breathing) is commonly seen in patients with diabetic ketoacidosis, while Cheyne-Stokes respiration (cyclical pattern of increasing and decreasing tidal volume) can indicate heart failure or neurological issues.
3. **Temperature:**
    - Normal body temperature ranges between 36.1°C and 37.2°C (97°F to 99°F), though diurnal variations and age-related differences are normal. Fever (temperature ≥ 38.0°C or 100.4°F) is a common sign of infection, inflammation, or malignancy. Conversely, hypothermia (temperature < 35.0°C or 95°F) may be indicative of sepsis, hypothyroidism, or environmental exposure.
    - In pediatrics, febrile illnesses are common, and accurate temperature measurement (preferably via a rectal thermometer for infants and young children) is crucial for proper diagnosis.
4. **Oxygen Saturation (SpO2):**
    - Pulse oximetry is a non-invasive way to measure peripheral oxygen saturation, and normal values range from 95-100%. Hypoxemia (SpO2 < 90%) can indicate respiratory or cardiovascular compromise, such as in cases of pneumonia, pulmonary embolism, or heart failure. Pulse oximetry is a valuable tool in assessing the severity of respiratory conditions and determining the need for supplemental oxygen.
    - Conditions like chronic obstructive pulmonary disease (COPD) may present with lower baseline SpO2 levels (88-92%), and interpretation of oxygen saturation in these cases requires clinical context.

C. Orthostatic Hypotension Assessment

Orthostatic hypotension is defined as a significant drop in blood pressure (usually ≥ 20 mmHg systolic or ≥ 10 mmHg diastolic) upon standing from a seated or supine position. It is a common cause of dizziness and falls in elderly patients but can affect younger individuals with certain conditions, such as dehydration, autonomic dysfunction, or medication side effects (e.g., antihypertensives, diuretics) .

1. **Procedure for Orthostatic BP Measurement:**
   - Measure BP and pulse after the patient has been lying down for at least 5 minutes.
   - Repeat measurements after the patient stands up for 1 minute, and again after 3 minutes.
   - A significant drop in BP or increase in pulse may indicate hypovolemia, autonomic dysfunction, or medication effects .

Orthostatic hypotension has been associated with increased morbidity and mortality, particularly in elderly populations, and should not be overlooked during the physical exam .

E. General Appearance

The general appearance of the patient provides critical clues that can guide further examination and diagnosis. Observing a patient's demeanor, posture, body habitus, and overall health status is often the first step in identifying potential underlying medical conditions.

1. Patient Demeanor:
   - A patient's level of alertness, interaction, and mood may indicate overall well-being or suggest underlying neurological or psychiatric issues. Lethargy or altered mental status can suggest infections like sepsis, metabolic disturbances, or intoxications, while an anxious or agitated demeanor may point toward respiratory distress or cardiac events such as a myocardial infarction .
2. Posture and Mobility:
   - Observing how a patient sits, stands, and moves can provide information about musculoskeletal or neurological impairments. For example, guarding or stiffness may suggest pain, while a stooped posture may be a sign of conditions like Parkinson's disease or advanced osteoarthritis. An unsteady gait could suggest cerebellar disease or peripheral neuropathy .
3. Body Habitus:
   - Body habitus offers important information regarding the patient's overall nutritional status and risk for chronic diseases. Obesity (especially central obesity) is a significant risk factor for conditions such as type 2 diabetes, hypertension, and cardiovascular disease. Conversely, cachexia or wasting may suggest chronic illness, malignancy, or malnutrition .
4. Recognizing Signs of Acute Distress:
   - Respiratory distress: Patients may exhibit increased work of breathing, accessory muscle use, or cyanosis. Labored breathing, tachypnea, or tripoding (leaning

forward with hands on knees) may suggest acute conditions such as asthma, pneumonia, or pulmonary edema .
- Cardiac distress: Patients with acute myocardial infarction or heart failure may appear pale, diaphoretic, or clutching their chest. An immediate assessment is needed in such cases to confirm the diagnosis and initiate treatment .
- Pain or discomfort: Non-verbal cues like grimacing, guarding, or restlessness can indicate underlying pain or distress that may require urgent intervention .

References

- Pickering, T. G., et al. "Recommendations for Blood Pressure Measurement in Humans and Experimental Animals." *Hypertension*, 2005.
- Verghese, A., et al. "The Physical Examination and the Fifth Vital Sign: The Value of Pulse Oximetry in Clinical Practice." *Journal of General Internal Medicine*, 2016.
- Epstein, R. M., et al. "Patient-Centered Communication: The Use of Physical Signs to Build Trust." *American Journal of Medicine*, 2008.
- Lipsitz, L. A. "Orthostatic Hypotension in the Elderly." *New England Journal of Medicine*, 2002.
- Bickley, L. S. "Bates' Guide to Physical Examination and History Taking." 13th ed., Wolters Kluwer, 2021.
- Marik, P. E. "Evaluation of Hypoxemia and Oxygen Therapy." *Chest*, 2015.
- Benarroch, E. "Neurogenic Orthostatic Hypotension: Pathophysiology and Management." *Neurology*, 2012.

Chapter 13. Head, Eyes, Ears, Nose, and Throat (HEENT) Examination

A. **Head and Scalp**

1. **Examining for Signs of Trauma, Tenderness, or Deformity**:
   - The examination of the **head and scalp** is essential for detecting abnormalities that may indicate trauma, congenital deformities, or systemic diseases. Begin by inspecting the **scalp** for visible lacerations, hematomas, or deformities, and palpate gently to assess for **tenderness** or **crepitus**, which could suggest underlying skull fractures .
   - **Scalp tenderness** may be a sign of conditions such as **temporal arteritis** (particularly in older adults), **trauma**, or **trigeminal neuralgia** . Temporal arteritis, a vasculitis that can cause scalp tenderness, is a serious condition that may lead to blindness if not promptly diagnosed and treated with corticosteroids.
   - **Deformities** of the skull can be congenital (e.g., **craniosynostosis** in infants) or acquired, such as from trauma. Observing the **size and shape of the skull** may reveal conditions like **hydrocephalus** in children or **Paget's disease** of the bone in older adults .

B. **Eyes**

1. **Visual Acuity Testing**:
   - **Visual acuity** is the most critical part of the eye examination and is typically assessed using a **Snellen chart** or near-vision card. Visual acuity should be measured with the patient's corrective lenses (if applicable), and results are documented in fraction form, with **20/20** being normal vision. Vision loss can result from refractive errors (e.g., myopia, hyperopia), cataracts, or retinal pathology such as **macular degeneration** .
   - For patients presenting with acute vision changes or loss, urgent referral for further ophthalmologic evaluation is necessary, as conditions such as **retinal detachment** or **acute angle-closure glaucoma** can lead to permanent vision loss if not treated promptly .
2. **Pupil Examination**:
   - The **pupils** should be assessed for **size, shape,** and **reactivity to light**. A normal pupil size ranges between 2-4 mm in bright light and 4-8 mm in dim light . The **pupillary light reflex** involves observing both **direct** and **consensual** responses to light. An abnormal response could indicate an issue with cranial nerve II (optic nerve) or III (oculomotor nerve).
   - **Anisocoria** (unequal pupil sizes) can be a normal variant in some individuals, but if it is new or associated with other neurological signs, it may indicate serious conditions such as **Horner's syndrome** (which presents with ptosis and anhidrosis) or **third nerve palsy** (which often presents with diplopia and ptosis) .
3. **Fundoscopic Examination**:

- **Fundoscopy** allows for the inspection of the **retina, optic disc, blood vessels**, and **macula**, providing a window into systemic diseases like hypertension, diabetes, and elevated intracranial pressure.
- Key findings include:
    - **Papilledema**, indicating increased intracranial pressure, manifests as swelling of the optic disc with blurred margins .
    - **Cotton-wool spots** and **hemorrhages** may indicate hypertensive retinopathy, while **microaneurysms** are typical in diabetic retinopathy .
- In elderly patients, **age-related macular degeneration** presents as **drusen** (yellow deposits beneath the retina), which are associated with central vision loss .

4. **Assessing for Jaundice, Pallor, and Conjunctival Abnormalities**:
    - **Jaundice** can be observed in the **sclera** (the white part of the eye), which often takes on a yellow hue in conditions such as **liver disease** (e.g., cirrhosis, hepatitis) or **hemolysis**.
    - **Pallor** of the conjunctiva may suggest **anemia**. A simple inspection by pulling down the lower eyelid can reveal whether the conjunctiva appears pale, a common finding in patients with hemoglobin levels below 8 g/dL .
    - **Conjunctival abnormalities**, such as **injection** (redness), may indicate conjunctivitis, while **subconjunctival hemorrhages** are often benign and can result from minor trauma or increased venous pressure (e.g., coughing or sneezing).

C. Ears

1. **Otoscopic Examination**:
    - The **otoscopic examination** is crucial for evaluating the **external auditory canal** and **tympanic membrane (TM)**. Begin by inspecting the ear canal for any signs of **obstruction** (e.g., cerumen impaction), **discharge**, or **foreign bodies** .
    - **Tympanic membrane** examination should include assessing for the color, position, and integrity of the membrane. A normal TM is pearly gray and translucent. Common abnormal findings include:
        - **Otitis media**: The TM may appear red and bulging with fluid behind it.
        - **Tympanic membrane perforation**: A visible hole in the TM, often resulting from trauma or chronic ear infections.
        - **Cholesteatoma**: A destructive lesion in the middle ear, often seen as a white mass, which can cause hearing loss and, if untreated, lead to serious complications .
2. **Hearing Assessment Techniques**:
    - **Whisper test**: Ask the patient to cover one ear while you whisper a combination of numbers and letters from 1-2 feet away. The patient should repeat what they hear.

- **Tuning fork tests**: The **Rinne test** and **Weber test** are used to differentiate between **conductive** and **sensorineural hearing loss**.
  - In the **Rinne test**, place a vibrating tuning fork on the patient's mastoid process and ask them to indicate when the sound stops. Then move the fork next to the ear canal. In normal hearing or sensorineural hearing loss, air conduction (AC) is better than bone conduction (BC). In conductive hearing loss, BC is greater than AC.
  - The **Weber test** involves placing a vibrating tuning fork on the patient's forehead. In **sensorineural hearing loss**, the sound lateralizes to the unaffected ear, while in **conductive hearing loss**, the sound lateralizes to the affected ear.

D. Nose and Sinuses

1. **Examining for Nasal Discharge, Septal Deviation, and Sinus Tenderness**:
   - **Nasal discharge** can be a clue to both infectious and allergic conditions. **Clear, watery discharge** is commonly seen in allergic rhinitis, whereas **thick, yellow-green discharge** may indicate bacterial sinusitis or infection. A **unilateral, foul-smelling discharge** in children may suggest a foreign body in the nostril.
   - Inspect the **nasal septum** for deviation, perforation, or evidence of trauma. A deviated septum is common and may contribute to nasal obstruction and recurrent sinusitis.
   - **Sinus tenderness** is assessed by palpating and lightly tapping over the **frontal** and **maxillary sinuses**. Tenderness suggests sinus inflammation or infection, particularly in cases of sinusitis. Additionally, transillumination of the sinuses can help assess for fluid accumulation in cases of suspected sinusitis.

E. Throat and Mouth

1. **Examining the Oral Mucosa, Pharynx, and Tonsils for Lesions, Erythema, or Exudates**:
   - Begin by inspecting the **oral mucosa** for any abnormalities, including **ulcers** (e.g., aphthous ulcers or oral thrush), **lesions** (e.g., leukoplakia, which can be precancerous), or **erythema**, which may suggest infection or inflammation. In patients with immunosuppression, oral lesions may be indicative of systemic diseases such as HIV or malignancies like Kaposi's sarcoma.
   - The **pharynx** and **tonsils** should be examined for **erythema, exudates**, or **swelling**. Erythematous and swollen tonsils with **white exudates** suggest bacterial infections like **streptococcal pharyngitis**, while a **grayish membrane** may be indicative of diphtheria, although rare.

- **Tonsillar hypertrophy** or asymmetry may suggest chronic tonsillitis or, in rare cases, a peritonsillar abscess. In cases of airway obstruction, such as seen in severe tonsillar hypertrophy, further evaluation or referral may be necessary.

References

- McGee, S. "Evidence-Based Physical Diagnosis." 4th ed., Elsevier, 2017.
- Bradley, P., et al. "Diagnostic Accuracy of the Otoscopic Examination for Acute Otitis Media: A Meta-Analysis." *Pediatrics*, 2016.
- Verghese, A. "The Physical Examination and Its Role in Clinical Diagnosis." *BMJ*, 2011.
- Munjal, V., et al. "Conductive and Sensorineural Hearing Loss in Otosclerosis: A Study Using Tuning Fork Tests." *Journal of Audiology and Otology*, 2018.
- Li, J. T., et al. "Sinusitis: Diagnosis and Treatment." *Mayo Clinic Proceedings*, 2015.
- Stevens, G., et al. "Chronic Tonsillitis and Adenotonsillar Hypertrophy in Children." *New England Journal of Medicine*, 2018.
- Solomon, D., et al. "Fundoscopy in Systemic Disease: A Window to Diagnosis." *American Journal of Medicine*, 2019.

Chapter 14. Neck Examination

A. Thyroid Examination

1. **Inspection and Palpation for Goiter, Nodules, or Tenderness**:
    - The thyroid gland plays a central role in regulating metabolism, and its enlargement or abnormality can signal a variety of systemic diseases, from hyperthyroidism to malignancy. A thorough thyroid examination begins with **inspection**, followed by **palpation**.
    - **Inspection**: Start by inspecting the neck for visible enlargement or asymmetry while the patient is seated and their neck slightly extended. Ask the patient to swallow while you observe the thyroid area. A **goiter** (enlarged thyroid gland) may become more apparent during swallowing, especially in conditions like **Graves' disease** or **iodine deficiency**. Symmetrical enlargement is commonly seen in diffuse goiters, while asymmetry may suggest nodules .
    - **Palpation**: After inspection, palpate the thyroid gland from behind the patient while they remain seated. Place your fingers on either side of the trachea, just below the cricoid cartilage, and ask the patient to swallow again. This technique helps distinguish between a diffuse goiter and a solitary nodule.
        - **Thyroid nodules**: Nodules are palpable lumps within the thyroid gland and can be solitary or multiple. Solitary nodules raise the concern of **thyroid cancer**, particularly in younger patients or those with a family history of thyroid malignancies. Nodules larger than 1 cm in diameter, irregular, or hard in texture should prompt further investigation with ultrasound or fine needle aspiration .
        - **Tenderness**: Palpation for tenderness is important in identifying **thyroiditis**, an inflammation of the thyroid gland. **Subacute (de Quervain's) thyroiditis** typically presents with a tender, enlarged thyroid and is often preceded by a viral infection. This condition can lead to transient hyperthyroidism, followed by hypothyroidism .
    - A **bruit** over the thyroid gland may be heard in patients with **Graves' disease** due to increased vascularity. This is usually assessed using a stethoscope.

B. Lymph Nodes

1. **Palpating Cervical, Supraclavicular, and Submandibular Nodes**:
    - Lymph node palpation is critical for detecting **lymphadenopathy**, which can indicate infections, malignancies, or systemic diseases like autoimmune disorders.
    - **Cervical lymph nodes**: Palpate the anterior and posterior cervical chains along the sternocleidomastoid muscle, feeling for size, tenderness, consistency, and mobility. **Acute infections**, such as streptococcal pharyngitis or mononucleosis, often result in tender, mobile lymph nodes, while firm, non-tender, and fixed

lymph nodes raise concern for malignancies such as **lymphoma** or **metastatic cancer**.
- **Submandibular nodes**: These nodes are located beneath the jaw and are commonly involved in infections of the mouth, teeth, or throat. Enlargement may be seen in cases of dental abscesses or submandibular gland infections.
- **Supraclavicular nodes**: Palpating the supraclavicular fossa is crucial for detecting more sinister causes of lymphadenopathy. The **Virchow's node** (left supraclavicular node) is particularly concerning for metastasis from intra-abdominal or thoracic malignancies (e.g., **gastric cancer**) and should always prompt further investigation if enlarged or firm.

2. **Recognizing Abnormal Lymphadenopathy**:
    - **Infectious lymphadenopathy** is typically soft, tender, and mobile. In contrast, **malignant nodes** tend to be hard, fixed to surrounding tissues, and non-tender. Enlarged lymph nodes larger than 1 cm, particularly if they persist for more than 4-6 weeks, should be evaluated with imaging (e.g., ultrasound or CT) and possibly a biopsy.
    - **Generalized lymphadenopathy**, involving multiple regions, can be seen in systemic illnesses like **HIV**, **sarcoidosis**, or **leukemia**.

C. **Jugular Venous Pressure (JVP)**

1. **Technique for Assessing JVP**:
    - Assessing the **jugular venous pressure (JVP)** is an essential part of the physical exam for evaluating right heart function and diagnosing conditions like **heart failure**. The JVP reflects the pressure in the right atrium and provides indirect evidence of central venous pressure (CVP).
    - **Technique**:
        - Position the patient at a **30-45 degree angle** (semi-recumbent) on the exam table. The head should be slightly turned to the left to allow better visualization of the right jugular vein.
        - Use tangential lighting to enhance visualization of the **internal jugular vein**, located just lateral to the sternocleidomastoid muscle. The **external jugular vein** can also be observed but may be less reliable due to valvular incompetence.
        - Measure the JVP by identifying the highest point of pulsation in the internal jugular vein. Using a ruler, align one edge at the sternal angle (Angle of Louis) and measure vertically to the level of venous pulsation. Normal JVP is **less than 3 cm above the sternal angle**.
        - A JVP measurement greater than 3 cm suggests elevated right atrial pressure and may indicate **congestive heart failure**, **constrictive pericarditis**, or **fluid overload**.
2. **Significance of Elevated JVP in Heart Failure**:

- **Elevated JVP** is a hallmark of **right-sided heart failure** or **biventricular heart failure**, where elevated pressures in the right atrium cause the jugular veins to become distended. This is often accompanied by other signs of heart failure such as **peripheral edema**, **hepatojugular reflux**, and **pulmonary crackles** .
- In **tricuspid regurgitation**, a systolic wave may be seen in the JVP waveform due to backward flow of blood from the right ventricle into the right atrium during systole.
- **Kussmaul's sign** (a paradoxical rise in JVP with inspiration) is seen in conditions like **constrictive pericarditis** and **right ventricular failure**, further highlighting the importance of JVP assessment in clinical diagnosis .

References

- Ross, D. S. "Evaluation and Treatment of Thyroid Nodules." *New England Journal of Medicine*, 2016.
- Bickley, L. S. "Bates' Guide to Physical Examination and History Taking." 13th ed., Wolters Kluwer, 2021.
- MacDonald, S., et al. "Lymphadenopathy: Differentiating Benign from Malignant Causes." *BMJ*, 2014.
- Marik, P. E. "Assessment of the Right Ventricular Function and Jugular Venous Pressure." *Critical Care Medicine*, 2016.
- Schrier, R. W., et al. "Mechanisms of Disease: Heart Failure and Volume Overload." *New England Journal of Medicine*, 2018.
- Stone, M. J., et al. "Clinical Approach to Lymphadenopathy and Splenomegaly." *Hematology/Oncology Clinics of North America*, 2017.
- Martin, T. J., et al. "Evaluation of Jugular Venous Pressure in the Diagnosis of Heart Failure." *American Journal of Cardiology*, 2015.

Chapter 15. Cardiovascular Examination

A. Inspection and Palpation

1. **Observing for Precordial Movement, Scars, or Deformities**:
    - **Precordial inspection** involves observing the anterior chest wall for visible movements or abnormalities. Significant **precordial movement** may suggest underlying heart disease, such as an enlarged heart (cardiomegaly) or **right ventricular hypertrophy**. Specifically, a **heave or lift** felt under the hand placed on the chest may indicate ventricular hypertrophy, while a **thrill** is a palpable vibration associated with turbulent blood flow, often overlying a significant murmur.
    - Inspect the chest for any **scars** that may indicate previous surgeries, such as coronary artery bypass grafting (CABG) or valve replacements. The presence of scars can provide critical historical context for the patient's cardiac history.
    - **Deformities** such as **pectus excavatum** (a sunken chest) can alter the heart's position and make auscultation more difficult. These anatomical variations should be noted during inspection.
2. **Palpating the Point of Maximal Impulse (PMI)**:
    - The **point of maximal impulse (PMI)** is the area where the cardiac impulse is most strongly felt, typically in the left 5th intercostal space at the midclavicular line. A displaced PMI (lateral or inferior) can be a sign of **left ventricular hypertrophy** (LVH) or cardiomegaly, often seen in conditions like **chronic hypertension** or **aortic stenosis**.
    - If the PMI is **sustained** or **forceful**, this may suggest left ventricular hypertrophy, while a **weak or absent** PMI could indicate conditions such as pericardial effusion or dilated cardiomyopathy. A normal PMI is typically a short, brisk tap, but alterations in character can point to underlying cardiac pathology.
    - **Palpation for thrills**: Thrills are palpable vibrations caused by turbulent blood flow and are usually associated with significant murmurs (e.g., aortic stenosis or ventricular septal defect). These are best palpated in areas where the murmur is loudest.

B. Auscultation

1. **Systematic Approach to Listening for Heart Sounds, Murmurs, and Rubs**:
    - A **systematic approach** to cardiac auscultation involves listening to the four primary areas:
        - **Aortic area** – 2nd right intercostal space.
        - **Pulmonic area** – 2nd left intercostal space.
        - **Tricuspid area** – 4th left intercostal space.
        - **Mitral area** – 5th left intercostal space at the midclavicular line (PMI).

- Use both the **diaphragm** and **bell** of the stethoscope. The **diaphragm** is best for high-pitched sounds (S1, S2, and most murmurs), while the **bell** is better for detecting low-pitched sounds (e.g., S3, S4, and certain murmurs like mitral stenosis).
- Instruct the patient to breathe normally, and listen during both inspiration and expiration, as some heart sounds or murmurs may change with respiration.

2. **Differentiating Between Normal and Abnormal Heart Sounds:**
    - **Normal heart sounds:**
        - **S1**: The first heart sound, caused by the closure of the mitral and tricuspid valves. It is best heard at the **apex** and marks the beginning of systole.
        - **S2**: The second heart sound, caused by the closure of the aortic and pulmonic valves. It is best heard at the **base** of the heart and marks the beginning of diastole. **Splitting of S2** during inspiration is normal, but persistent splitting during both inspiration and expiration may suggest right bundle branch block or pulmonary hypertension.
    - **Abnormal heart sounds:**
        - **S3**: Also called a **ventricular gallop**, S3 can indicate volume overload states such as **heart failure**. It is heard just after S2 and is best detected at the **apex** with the bell.
        - **S4**: Also called an **atrial gallop**, S4 is associated with a stiff or hypertrophic ventricle, often due to **hypertension**, **aortic stenosis**, or ischemic heart disease. It is heard just before S1.
        - **Murmurs**: These are caused by turbulent blood flow and may signify valvular disease. **Systolic murmurs** (e.g., **aortic stenosis**, **mitral regurgitation**) occur between S1 and S2, while **diastolic murmurs** (e.g., **aortic regurgitation**, **mitral stenosis**) occur between S2 and the next S1.
        - **Pericardial rubs**: A **friction rub** is a high-pitched, scratchy sound that is best heard with the diaphragm at the left lower sternal border. It is caused by inflamed pericardial layers rubbing against each other, often due to **pericarditis**.

C. Peripheral Vascular Exam

1. **Palpating Pulses, Assessing for Bruits, and Evaluating Capillary Refill:**
    - The **peripheral vascular examination** involves palpating the pulses, assessing for bruits (indicative of turbulent blood flow), and checking capillary refill to assess perfusion.
    - **Palpating pulses**: Assess the **carotid, brachial, radial, femoral, popliteal, posterior tibial, and dorsalis pedis** pulses bilaterally. Normal pulses should be strong and equal bilaterally. A **weak or absent pulse** may indicate **peripheral arterial disease** (PAD), while a **bounding pulse** may suggest hyperdynamic circulation as seen in conditions like **aortic regurgitation**.

- **Assessing for bruits**: Bruits are audible sounds caused by turbulent blood flow through a narrowed artery. To assess for **carotid bruits**, use the **bell** of the stethoscope and ask the patient to hold their breath while you listen along the carotid artery. Carotid bruits may indicate **carotid artery stenosis**, which increases the risk of stroke .
    - **Capillary refill**: This is a simple test to assess peripheral perfusion. Press on the nail bed or the pad of a finger or toe until it blanches, and then release. Normal refill time is less than **2 seconds**. A delayed refill (>2 seconds) may indicate **shock**, **dehydration**, or peripheral vascular disease .
2. **Examining for Signs of Venous Insufficiency or Arterial Disease**:
    - **Venous insufficiency**: Look for signs such as **varicose veins**, **pitting edema**, **skin discoloration**, or **ulceration**. Patients with chronic venous insufficiency may develop **stasis dermatitis** (brownish discoloration around the ankles) and **venous ulcers** on the medial malleolus .
    - **Arterial disease**: Signs of **peripheral arterial disease (PAD)** include **pallor**, **cool extremities**, **diminished pulses**, and **non-healing ulcers**. In severe cases, **gangrene** may develop. The **ankle-brachial index (ABI)** is a non-invasive test used to assess for PAD and involves comparing the blood pressure in the ankle to that in the arm. An ABI less than **0.90** suggests PAD .
    - **Edema**: **Bilateral pitting edema** is often seen in conditions such as **heart failure**, **kidney disease**, or **venous insufficiency**. Unilateral edema may indicate **deep vein thrombosis (DVT)** and warrants urgent investigation.

References

- Bickley, L. S. "Bates' Guide to Physical Examination and History Taking." 13th ed., Wolters Kluwer, 2021.
- McGee, S. "Evidence-Based Physical Diagnosis." 4th ed., Elsevier, 2017.
- Nishimura, R. A., et al. "2017 AHA/ACC Focused Update of the 2014 AHA/ACC Guideline for the Management of Patients with Valvular Heart Disease." *Journal of the American College of Cardiology*, 2017.
- Moran, J. E., et al. "Clinical Approach to the Patient with Lower Extremity Peripheral Arterial Disease." *New England Journal of Medicine*, 2018.
- Marik, P. E., et al. "Pericardial Diseases: Diagnosis and Management." *New England Journal of Medicine*, 2019.
- Aboyans, V., et al. "Measurement and Interpretation of the Ankle-Brachial Index: A Scientific Statement from the American Heart Association." *Circulation*, 2012.

Chapter 16. Respiratory Examination

A. Inspection

1. **Assessing Respiratory Rate, Pattern, and Effort**:
   - **Respiratory rate** is the number of breaths a patient takes per minute, and it provides critical insight into the patient's respiratory and overall health. The normal respiratory rate for adults is **12-20 breaths per minute**. Tachypnea (a rapid respiratory rate) may indicate conditions such as **pneumonia, pulmonary embolism**, or **metabolic acidosis**, while bradypnea (a slow rate) can be seen in **CNS depression** or **opioid overdose** .
   - **Respiratory pattern** and effort are key to evaluating the patient's work of breathing. Observe patterns such as **Kussmaul breathing**, which is deep, rapid breathing often associated with **diabetic ketoacidosis**, or **Cheyne-Stokes respiration**, a cyclic pattern of breathing associated with **heart failure** or **neurological disorders** . **Paradoxical breathing** (inward movement of the abdomen during inspiration) can suggest diaphragm dysfunction or **respiratory muscle fatigue**.
   - Assess for signs of increased **respiratory effort**, such as the use of **accessory muscles** (sternocleidomastoid, scalene muscles), **nasal flaring**, and **tracheal tugging**. These findings are often seen in patients with severe respiratory distress due to conditions such as **COPD, asthma**, or **pneumothorax**.
2. **Observing for Chest Wall Deformities or Use of Accessory Muscles**:
   - Structural abnormalities of the chest wall, such as **pectus excavatum** (sunken chest) or **pectus carinatum** (protruding chest), can affect respiratory function by reducing lung expansion. These deformities may be congenital or acquired and can lead to **restrictive lung disease** if severe .
   - **Barrel chest**, which is an increased anterior-posterior diameter of the chest, is commonly seen in patients with **chronic obstructive pulmonary disease (COPD)**, where chronic hyperinflation of the lungs results in altered chest shape.
   - **Use of accessory muscles** (e.g., sternocleidomastoid, intercostal muscles) during breathing often indicates increased respiratory effort and is a sign of **respiratory distress** in conditions like **acute asthma exacerbation** or **pulmonary edema**.

B. Palpation and Percussion

1. **Palpating for Tenderness, Chest Expansion, and Tactile Fremitus**:
   - **Palpation for tenderness**: Gently palpate the chest wall for any areas of tenderness, which can indicate **rib fractures, pleurisy**, or **costochondritis** (inflammation of the cartilage connecting the ribs to the sternum) . In patients

with trauma or recent surgery, localized tenderness may suggest complications like pneumothorax or rib contusions.
- **Chest expansion**: Place your hands on the patient's back at the level of the 10th ribs with your thumbs meeting at the midline. Ask the patient to take a deep breath, and observe the movement of your hands. In healthy individuals, both sides of the chest should expand symmetrically. **Asymmetric chest expansion** may suggest **unilateral pneumonia, pleural effusion**, or **pneumothorax**.
- **Tactile fremitus**: This is the vibration felt on the chest wall when the patient speaks. To assess, place the ulnar edge of your hand or fingertips on the patient's chest and ask them to say "ninety-nine." Increased tactile fremitus can indicate **consolidation** (as seen in pneumonia), while decreased fremitus suggests conditions like **pleural effusion, pneumothorax**, or **obstructed bronchus**.

2. **Percussing for Areas of Dullness or Hyperresonance**:
   - Percussion involves tapping on the chest wall to detect differences in resonance. **Normal lung tissue** produces a resonant sound, while deviations from this indicate underlying pathology.
   - **Dullness to percussion**: This suggests **consolidation, pleural effusion**, or **atelectasis**. For example, dullness over the base of the lung is a classic sign of pleural effusion.
   - **Hyperresonance**: This is a hollow sound that indicates increased air within the thorax, commonly seen in conditions like **pneumothorax** or **emphysema**. **Bilateral hyperresonance** may suggest COPD, while **unilateral hyperresonance** could indicate a large pneumothorax or severe bullous disease.

C. Auscultation

1. **Recognizing Normal Breath Sounds and Differentiating Abnormal Sounds**:
   - Auscultation is the most critical component of the respiratory exam and should be done systematically. Listen to the **anterior, posterior, and lateral** chest, instructing the patient to breathe deeply through the mouth.
   - **Normal breath sounds**:
     - **Vesicular breath sounds**: These are soft, low-pitched sounds heard over most of the lung fields and represent normal air movement.
     - **Bronchial breath sounds**: These are louder, higher-pitched sounds heard over the large airways (trachea and bronchi). Bronchial breath sounds heard in the periphery may suggest **lung consolidation** (e.g., pneumonia).
   - **Abnormal breath sounds**:
     - **Crackles (rales)**: These are discontinuous sounds, often likened to the sound of popping or crackling. They are associated with conditions such

as **pneumonia**, **pulmonary edema** (e.g., heart failure), or **interstitial lung disease**. Fine crackles suggest alveolar fluid or fibrosis, while coarse crackles indicate airway secretions.
- **Wheezes**: These are high-pitched, musical sounds caused by narrowed airways, typically heard in **asthma**, **COPD**, or **bronchitis**.
- **Rhonchi**: These are low-pitched, snoring sounds caused by secretions in the larger airways. They are often cleared with coughing and are commonly seen in **bronchitis**.
- **Pleural friction rub**: This is a low-pitched, grating sound heard when inflamed pleural surfaces rub against each other, often seen in **pleuritis** or **pleural effusion**. It is best heard during both inspiration and expiration over the affected area.

2. **Use of Voice Resonance Techniques**:
   - **Voice resonance tests** involve listening to the patient's spoken voice through the stethoscope to assess for lung pathology.
     - **Bronchophony**: Ask the patient to say "ninety-nine" while you auscultate the lung fields. In normal lungs, the sound is muffled. **Increased clarity** of the sound suggests **consolidation**, as sound is transmitted more effectively through solid or liquid-filled lung tissue.
     - **Egophony**: Ask the patient to say "E" while you listen with the stethoscope. In normal lungs, you will hear an "E" sound. However, if the "E" sounds like an "A," this suggests lung consolidation, as seen in **pneumonia**.
     - **Whispered pectoriloquy**: Ask the patient to whisper "ninety-nine." In normal lungs, the whispered sound should be faint or indistinct. If the whisper is heard clearly, it indicates consolidation or fibrosis.

References

- McGee, S. "Evidence-Based Physical Diagnosis." 4th ed., Elsevier, 2017.
- Bickley, L. S. "Bates' Guide to Physical Examination and History Taking." 13th ed., Wolters Kluwer, 2021.
- Bellani, G., et al. "Acute Respiratory Distress Syndrome." *JAMA*, 2016.
- Lee, W. Y., et al. "Clinical Approach to the Patient with Chronic Dyspnea." *New England Journal of Medicine*, 2018.
- Mendez-Tellez, P. A., et al. "Crackles and Wheezes: An Evidence-Based Approach." *Chest*, 2017.
- Noble, V. E., & Nelson, B. P. "Manual of Emergency and Critical Care Ultrasound." 2nd ed., Cambridge University Press, 2011.
- Lichtenstein, D. A. "Lung Ultrasound in the Critically Ill." *Annals of Intensive Care*, 2014.

Chapter 17. Gastrointestinal Examination

A. Inspection

1. **Observing for Abdominal Distention, Scars, or Skin Changes**:
   - **Abdominal distention** is an important visual clue that may indicate the presence of gas, fluid, or a mass within the abdominal cavity. Common causes of abdominal distention include **ascites, bowel obstruction**, and **organomegaly**. In cases of ascites, the abdomen may appear protuberant with bulging flanks, while a distended, tympanitic abdomen is suggestive of **bowel obstruction** or **paralytic ileus**.
   - **Scars** from previous surgeries provide valuable information about the patient's medical and surgical history. For example, scars from an appendectomy, cholecystectomy, or laparotomy can indicate past abdominal procedures. The location and type of scar (e.g., midline, transverse, or laparoscopic) help guide the differential diagnosis for the patient's current presentation.
   - **Skin changes** such as **striae** (stretch marks) can be seen in patients with recent rapid weight gain or **Cushing's syndrome**. **Caput medusae** (dilated superficial veins on the abdomen) may indicate **portal hypertension** due to **liver cirrhosis**. Other skin findings, such as **ecchymosis** in the flanks (**Grey-Turner sign**) or periumbilical area (**Cullen's sign**), can suggest intra-abdominal hemorrhage (e.g., **acute pancreatitis** or ruptured ectopic pregnancy).

B. Auscultation

1. **Listening for Bowel Sounds and Bruits**:
   - **Bowel sounds** are an important indicator of gastrointestinal function and should be auscultated with the diaphragm of the stethoscope before performing any palpation or percussion, as these maneuvers can alter bowel activity. Normal bowel sounds are intermittent and gurgling, occurring about 5-30 times per minute. **Hyperactive bowel sounds** can suggest **gastroenteritis, early bowel obstruction**, or **diarrhea**, while **hypoactive or absent bowel sounds** (after listening for at least 2 minutes) may indicate **ileus** or **peritonitis**.
   - **Bruits** are abnormal vascular sounds that may indicate turbulent blood flow through a vessel. Auscultate over the **aorta, renal arteries, iliac arteries**, and **femoral arteries** for bruits. **Aortic bruits** may suggest an **abdominal aortic aneurysm (AAA)**, while **renal bruits** could indicate **renal artery stenosis**, a common cause of secondary hypertension.

C. Percussion

1. **Percussing for Organomegaly and Abdominal Fluid**:
    - **Percussion** helps assess the presence of gas, fluid, or solid masses in the abdomen. In a healthy individual, the abdomen is mostly tympanic (due to gas in the intestines), with dullness over solid organs such as the liver and spleen.
    - **Liver span**: Percuss the liver span by starting at the midclavicular line below the nipple and working downward from the lung (resonant) to the liver (dull) and then continuing downward until bowel sounds return (tympanic). A normal liver span is typically **6-12 cm**. An enlarged liver (hepatomegaly) may be seen in **congestive heart failure, hepatitis**, or **fatty liver disease** .
    - **Spleen**: The spleen is normally not percussable unless enlarged. Percussion in the **Traube's space** (left lower anterior chest wall) is often used to assess for **splenomegaly**, which can occur in **hemolytic anemia, portal hypertension**, or **infections** like **mononucleosis**.
2. **Assessing for Shifting Dullness and Fluid Wave in Ascites**:
    - **Shifting dullness**: In cases of **ascites**, fluid collects in the dependent areas of the abdomen. To assess for shifting dullness, percuss from the midline of the abdomen to the flanks while the patient is supine. If dullness is present in the flanks, have the patient roll onto one side and repeat the percussion. A shift in the location of the dullness indicates free fluid in the abdomen, a hallmark of ascites .
    - **Fluid wave test**: This is another test for ascites. The patient places their hand firmly along the midline of their abdomen to prevent the transmission of movement through subcutaneous tissue. The examiner taps one flank while feeling for a wave on the opposite flank. The presence of a fluid wave suggests large-volume ascites, which is commonly seen in **liver cirrhosis, heart failure**, or **peritoneal carcinomatosis** .

D. Palpation

1. **Systematic Palpation for Tenderness, Masses, Hepatomegaly, and Splenomegaly**:
    - **Palpation** should always begin with light palpation, followed by deeper palpation to assess for tenderness, guarding, masses, or organomegaly.
    - **Tenderness**: Localized tenderness may suggest underlying inflammation or infection of the corresponding organ. For example, **epigastric tenderness** could indicate **peptic ulcer disease** or **gastritis**, while **right lower quadrant tenderness** is a classic finding in **acute appendicitis**.
    - **Masses**: Palpating for abdominal masses involves distinguishing between solid and cystic masses. A solid mass could indicate **tumors** (e.g., colorectal cancer, liver metastasis), while a fluid-filled mass could be a **cyst** or **abscess**.
    - **Hepatomegaly**: Palpate the liver edge by placing your hand just below the right costal margin while the patient takes a deep breath. A smooth, enlarged liver suggests **hepatic congestion** (due to heart failure), while a firm, nodular liver raises concern for **cirrhosis** or **liver cancer**.

- **Splenomegaly**: Begin palpation of the spleen in the right lower quadrant and move toward the left costal margin as the patient takes deep breaths. An enlarged spleen can indicate **portal hypertension**, **hematologic malignancies**, or **infectious mononucleosis**.
2. **Assessing for Guarding, Rebound Tenderness, and Murphy's Sign**:
    - **Guarding**: This is the involuntary tensing of the abdominal muscles in response to palpation and can be a sign of **peritonitis**. It may be localized or diffuse, depending on the extent of the inflammation.
    - **Rebound tenderness**: Rebound tenderness is elicited by pressing gently and deeply on the abdomen, then releasing the pressure quickly. If the patient experiences more pain upon release than during compression, it suggests **peritoneal irritation** (e.g., from **appendicitis**, **perforated ulcer**, or **diverticulitis**).
    - **Murphy's sign**: This is a specific test for **cholecystitis** (inflammation of the gallbladder). To perform this test, place your fingers under the right costal margin at the midclavicular line and ask the patient to take a deep breath. A positive **Murphy's sign** occurs when the patient suddenly stops inhaling due to pain, indicating gallbladder inflammation.

References

- McGee, S. "Evidence-Based Physical Diagnosis." 4th ed., Elsevier, 2017.
- Bickley, L. S. "Bates' Guide to Physical Examination and History Taking." 13th ed., Wolters Kluwer, 2021.
- Tarn, A. C., & Lapworth, R. "Abdominal Examination: Which Diagnostic Signs Are Valid?" *Postgraduate Medical Journal*, 2009.
- Trowbridge, R. L., et al. "Does This Patient Have Acute Cholecystitis? The Rational Clinical Examination." *JAMA*, 2003.
- Runyon, B. A. "Management of Adult Patients with Ascites Due to Cirrhosis: An Update." *Hepatology*, 2009.
- Sherlock, S., & Dooley, J. "Diseases of the Liver and Biliary System." 12th ed., Blackwell Science, 2011.
- Talley, N. J., & O'Connor, S. "Clinical Examination: A Systematic Guide to Physical Diagnosis." 8th ed., Elsevier, 2020.

Chapter 18. Musculoskeletal Examination

A. General Inspection

1. **Observing for Joint Deformities, Swelling, or Asymmetry**:
   - A thorough musculoskeletal exam begins with general inspection, focusing on the **symmetry** of the joints and surrounding structures. Inspect for any **deformities**, **swelling**, **muscle atrophy**, or **erythema** that could indicate underlying pathology.
   - **Joint deformities** are common in conditions such as **rheumatoid arthritis (RA)**, where chronic inflammation leads to **ulnar deviation** of the fingers, **swan neck** or **boutonniere deformities**. **Osteoarthritis** may present with **Heberden's nodes** (distal interphalangeal joint swelling) and **Bouchard's nodes** (proximal interphalangeal joint swelling).
   - **Swelling** may indicate **synovitis**, **effusion**, or **bursitis**. It is often associated with acute inflammatory processes like **gout**, **septic arthritis**, or **reactive arthritis**. Chronic joint swelling is a hallmark of conditions such as **osteoarthritis** or **rheumatoid arthritis**.
   - **Asymmetry** in joint size, shape, or range of motion may suggest **trauma**, **muscle imbalance**, or conditions such as **hemiplegia** from a stroke. In children, asymmetry could point to congenital issues such as **developmental dysplasia of the hip**.
2. **Assessing Gait and Range of Motion**:
   - **Gait analysis** provides essential clues about musculoskeletal and neurological integrity. Observe the patient walking and note any abnormalities such as **limping**, **antalgic gait** (shortened stance phase due to pain), or **Trendelenburg gait** (indicative of weak hip abductor muscles). **Ataxic gait** can suggest cerebellar dysfunction, while a **shuffling gait** may be seen in **Parkinson's disease**.
   - Assess **range of motion (ROM)** for all major joints, including active (patient-driven) and passive (examiner-assisted) movements. Reduced ROM may indicate joint stiffness from conditions like **osteoarthritis**, soft tissue injury, or muscle contractures.
     - For example, limited **shoulder abduction** can occur in **rotator cuff tears**, while reduced **hip flexion** may suggest **osteoarthritis** or **avascular necrosis**. Compare ROM bilaterally to detect asymmetries that may suggest a localized issue.

B. Joint-Specific Examination

1. **Detailed Examination of the Shoulders, Elbows, Wrists, Hands, Hips, Knees, Ankles, and Feet**:

- **Shoulder**: Assess the **glenohumeral joint** and **acromioclavicular joint** for tenderness, swelling, and deformity. Test ROM (flexion, abduction, internal and external rotation). Pain with abduction or external rotation may indicate **rotator cuff injury** or **impingement syndrome**.
- **Elbow**: Palpate for tenderness over the **medial epicondyle** (golfer's elbow) and **lateral epicondyle** (tennis elbow). Test for **flexion, extension, supination**, and **pronation**.
- **Wrist and Hands**: Assess for **deformities**, such as the **Z-thumb deformity** in rheumatoid arthritis or **Dupuytren's contracture** (palmar fascia thickening). Palpate for **tenderness**, especially at the **anatomic snuffbox**, which may indicate **scaphoid fracture**. Test **grip strength** and **wrist flexion/extension**.
- **Hips**: Palpate for tenderness in the **trochanteric bursa** and assess ROM (flexion, extension, abduction, and internal/external rotation). Limited internal rotation is often an early sign of **hip osteoarthritis**.
- **Knees**: Palpate the **patella, tibial tuberosity**, and **joint line** for tenderness. Effusion or swelling may indicate **ligament injuries, meniscal tears**, or **osteoarthritis**. Test ROM and perform special tests such as the **McMurray's test** (for meniscal tears) and **Lachman's test** (for anterior cruciate ligament injury).
- **Ankles and Feet**: Inspect for **swelling, deformities**, or **plantar fasciitis**. Assess ROM (dorsiflexion, plantarflexion, inversion, eversion). Palpate the **Achilles tendon** for tenderness or rupture. Swelling of the **metatarsophalangeal joint** may indicate **gout**.

2. **Special Maneuvers to Assess for Joint Stability and Inflammation**:
    - **Tinel's sign**: Tapping over the **median nerve** at the wrist may produce tingling in the fingers, indicating **carpal tunnel syndrome**.
    - **Phalen's test**: Flex the patient's wrists and hold for 30-60 seconds. Tingling in the distribution of the **median nerve** (thumb, index, middle fingers) suggests **carpal tunnel syndrome**.
    - **McMurray's test**: This maneuver evaluates the **menisci** of the knee. With the patient supine, flex the knee and rotate the tibia while extending the knee. A palpable click or pain may indicate a **meniscal tear**.
    - **Lachman's test**: Assess **anterior cruciate ligament (ACL) stability** by flexing the knee at 30 degrees and pulling the tibia anteriorly. An increased anterior translation of the tibia indicates **ACL tear**.

C. Spine Examination

1. **Assessing for Tenderness, Deformity, and Range of Motion**:
    - **Inspection**: Observe the alignment of the spine from both the front and side. Look for abnormal curves such as **kyphosis** (excessive thoracic curvature), **lordosis** (excessive lumbar curvature), or **scoliosis** (lateral curvature). These

deformities can result from conditions like **osteoporosis**, **degenerative disc disease**, or **congenital spine abnormalities** .
- **Palpation**: Palpate the **spinous processes**, **paraspinal muscles**, and **sacroiliac joints** for tenderness. Pain over the vertebral bodies may suggest a **vertebral fracture** or **infection**, while tenderness over the paraspinal muscles often indicates **muscle strain** or **spasm**.
- **Range of Motion**: Test ROM by asking the patient to **flex**, **extend**, **laterally bend**, and **rotate** the spine. Reduced ROM may be due to **degenerative disc disease**, **spinal stenosis**, or **ankylosing spondylitis**. Limited **lumbar flexion** with pain suggests **disc herniation** or **sciatica**.
- **Special Tests**:
  - **Straight leg raise**: This test evaluates for **lumbar disc herniation**. With the patient supine, raise the leg while keeping the knee extended. Pain radiating down the leg (especially below the knee) indicates a positive test, suggestive of **sciatica** or **nerve root compression**.
  - **Schober's test**: Used to assess the flexibility of the lumbar spine, particularly in **ankylosing spondylitis**. The patient stands upright, and the distance between two marked points on the lumbar spine is measured while the patient bends forward. A reduced increase in distance indicates restricted spinal mobility .

References

- McGee, S. "Evidence-Based Physical Diagnosis." 4th ed., Elsevier, 2017.
- Bickley, L. S. "Bates' Guide to Physical Examination and History Taking." 13th ed., Wolters Kluwer, 2021.
- American College of Rheumatology. "Guidelines for the Management of Rheumatoid Arthritis." *Arthritis Care & Research*, 2021.
- Neogi, T., et al. "2015 ACR-EULAR Classification Criteria for Gout." *Arthritis & Rheumatology*, 2015.
- Martin, G. M., et al. "Evaluation of the Knee: ACL and Meniscus Injuries." *Journal of Orthopaedic Surgery and Research*, 2016.
- Ropper, A. H., et al. "Lumbar Disc Herniation and Sciatica." *New England Journal of Medicine*, 2015.
- Ranganathan, P., et al. "Ankylosing Spondylitis: Clinical Features and Diagnostic Criteria." *Lancet*, 2017.

Chapter 19. Neurological Examination

A. **Mental Status and Cognitive Function**

1. **Assessing Orientation, Memory, and Higher Cognitive Functions**:
   - The mental status examination assesses a patient's **cognitive function**, which includes orientation, memory, attention, language, and higher-order cognitive abilities. This is crucial in diagnosing **dementia, delirium, stroke**, and other neurological or psychiatric conditions.
   - **Orientation** is evaluated by asking the patient about **person, place**, and **time** (e.g., "What is your name? Where are you? What is the date?"). Disorientation can be an early sign of **delirium, traumatic brain injury**, or **global cognitive decline**, such as in **Alzheimer's disease** .
   - **Memory** is assessed by testing both **short-term** and **long-term memory**. Ask the patient to recall a series of words immediately and again after a few minutes. Impairments in short-term memory can be seen in conditions like **amnesia** or **mild cognitive impairment**. Testing long-term memory involves asking about past events (e.g., historical events or personal milestones).
   - **Higher cognitive functions** include abilities such as **language, abstract reasoning**, and **executive function**. You can test **language** by asking the patient to name objects or repeat phrases. **Abstract reasoning** can be tested with tasks like interpreting proverbs or identifying similarities (e.g., "How are a bicycle and a car alike?"). Impairment in higher cognitive functions is seen in **frontotemporal dementia, stroke**, or **traumatic brain injury** .

B. **Cranial Nerve Examination**

1. **Detailed Assessment of All 12 Cranial Nerves**:
   - The **cranial nerve examination** is essential for detecting **localized brain lesions, neuropathies**, and conditions like **multiple sclerosis, stroke**, or **tumors**. Each nerve is responsible for specific sensory or motor functions:
     - **CN I (Olfactory nerve)**: Test by asking the patient to identify familiar odors (e.g., coffee or peppermint). **Anosmia** (loss of smell) can result from **head trauma, sinus disease**, or **neurodegenerative diseases** like **Parkinson's** or **Alzheimer's** .
     - **CN II (Optic nerve)**: Assess **visual acuity** with a Snellen chart, **visual fields** by confrontation, and the **fundoscopic exam** to observe the optic disc. **Optic neuritis** (inflammation of the optic nerve) is often an early sign of **multiple sclerosis** .
     - **CN III, IV, VI (Oculomotor, Trochlear, Abducens nerves)**: Test **pupil response to light** and **extraocular movements**. Assess for **ptosis** (drooping eyelid) or **diplopia** (double vision), which may indicate **nerve palsies** from **diabetes, aneurysms**, or **tumors**.

- **CN V (Trigeminal nerve)**: Test **sensation** over the face (ophthalmic, maxillary, mandibular branches) and the **corneal reflex**. Test **jaw strength** by asking the patient to clench their teeth. **Trigeminal neuralgia** causes severe, stabbing facial pain along the nerve's distribution.
- **CN VII (Facial nerve)**: Ask the patient to raise their eyebrows, close their eyes tightly, and smile. Asymmetry may indicate **Bell's palsy** (peripheral nerve lesion) or **stroke** (central lesion).
- **CN VIII (Vestibulocochlear nerve)**: Test **hearing** using the **Rinne** and **Weber tests** with a tuning fork. Assess **balance** for vestibular function. Hearing loss or vertigo may result from **acoustic neuroma**, **labyrinthitis**, or **Meniere's disease**.
- **CN IX, X (Glossopharyngeal and Vagus nerves)**: Check the **gag reflex** and assess the **soft palate** for symmetry when the patient says "ah." A unilateral deviation of the uvula may suggest a lesion in one of these nerves.
- **CN XI (Accessory nerve)**: Test **shoulder shrug** (trapezius) and **head turning** (sternocleidomastoid) against resistance. Weakness may suggest **nerve damage** from neck surgery or trauma.
- **CN XII (Hypoglossal nerve)**: Ask the patient to stick out their tongue and assess for **deviation** or **fasciculations**. A deviated tongue suggests a hypoglossal nerve lesion.

C. Motor and Sensory Function

1. **Testing Muscle Strength, Tone, and Bulk**:
   - **Muscle strength** is tested using the **Medical Research Council (MRC) grading scale** (0 to 5), with 5 being normal strength and 0 indicating no movement. Muscle weakness can be a sign of **upper motor neuron disease** (e.g., stroke, multiple sclerosis) or **lower motor neuron disease** (e.g., peripheral neuropathy, amyotrophic lateral sclerosis).
   - **Muscle tone** refers to the resistance felt during passive movement. **Spasticity** (increased tone) suggests an **upper motor neuron lesion** (e.g., stroke, multiple sclerosis), while **flaccidity** (decreased tone) indicates **lower motor neuron disease** (e.g., Guillain-Barré syndrome).
   - **Muscle bulk** should be symmetric. **Atrophy** may be a sign of **chronic lower motor neuron damage** or **muscle disease** such as **muscular dystrophy**.
2. **Sensory Testing for Light Touch, Pain, Vibration, and Proprioception**:
   - **Light touch** is tested using a cotton wisp, while **pain** sensation is assessed with a sharp object (e.g., a pin). Sensory loss may suggest **nerve root compression** or **diabetic neuropathy**.

- **Vibration sense** is tested using a 128 Hz tuning fork on the distal joints (e.g., fingers, toes). Loss of vibration sense is common in **peripheral neuropathy** (e.g., diabetes, vitamin B12 deficiency).
- **Proprioception** is tested by moving the patient's fingers or toes up and down and asking them to identify the direction. Loss of proprioception may suggest a lesion in the **posterior columns** of the spinal cord, seen in **tabes dorsalis** or **vitamin B12 deficiency**.

D. Reflexes

1. **Deep Tendon Reflexes, Babinski's Sign, and Clonus**:
   - **Deep tendon reflexes (DTRs)** are tested using a reflex hammer, and they are graded on a scale of 0 to 4+ (2+ is normal). **Hyperreflexia** (increased reflexes) suggests **upper motor neuron lesions** (e.g., stroke, multiple sclerosis), while **hyporeflexia** (decreased reflexes) suggests **lower motor neuron disease** (e.g., peripheral neuropathy, spinal cord injury).
   - The **Babinski sign** is tested by stroking the lateral aspect of the foot's sole. A normal response is **toe flexion**, but **dorsiflexion** of the great toe (positive Babinski sign) suggests **corticospinal tract damage** (e.g., from stroke or trauma).
   - **Clonus** refers to rhythmic, involuntary muscle contractions after a sudden stretch and indicates **upper motor neuron disease**. Clonus is often tested by briskly dorsiflexing the foot; repeated jerking movements suggest **spinal cord pathology**.

E. Coordination and Gait

1. **Assessing Cerebellar Function with Tests such as Romberg, Finger-to-Nose, and Heel-to-Shin**:
   - **Romberg test**: This test assesses **proprioception** and **balance**. Ask the patient to stand with feet together and eyes closed. Swaying or falling suggests **sensory ataxia**, often due to posterior column disease (e.g., **vitamin B12 deficiency, tabes dorsalis**). A positive Romberg test may indicate **sensory ataxia**, whereas cerebellar ataxia is present even with eyes open.
   - **Finger-to-nose test**: Ask the patient to touch their nose and then touch the examiner's finger repeatedly. **Dysmetria** (overshooting or undershooting the target) suggests **cerebellar dysfunction**.
   - **Heel-to-shin test**: The patient slides the heel of one foot down the opposite shin. Difficulty performing this test also suggests **cerebellar disease** (e.g., **stroke, multiple sclerosis, alcohol intoxication**).
2. **Observing Gait and Balance**:

- Gait assessment helps detect abnormalities in **motor strength**, **coordination**, and **balance**. Common gait abnormalities include:
    - **Ataxic gait**: Wide-based, unsteady gait seen in **cerebellar dysfunction** (e.g., cerebellar stroke, multiple sclerosis).
    - **Parkinsonian gait**: Shuffling steps with reduced arm swing and forward-leaning posture, characteristic of **Parkinson's disease**.
    - **Steppage gait**: High stepping due to foot drop, often seen in **peripheral neuropathy** or **lumbar disc herniation**.
- **Tandem gait** (walking heel-to-toe in a straight line) assesses cerebellar function and balance.

References

- McGee, S. "Evidence-Based Physical Diagnosis." 4th ed., Elsevier, 2017.
- Bickley, L. S. "Bates' Guide to Physical Examination and History Taking." 13th ed., Wolters Kluwer, 2021.
- Campbell, W. W., et al. "Evaluation and Management of Peripheral Nerve Disorders." *New England Journal of Medicine*, 2018.
- Goldman, L., et al. "Cranial Nerve Palsies in Neurological Disease." *Journal of Neurology*, 2020.
- Kandel, E. R., et al. "Neurological Reflexes and Gait: Clinical Assessment and Pathophysiology." *Journal of Clinical Neurology*, 2019.
- Román, G. C. "Neurological Complications of Vitamin B12 Deficiency." *Lancet Neurology*, 2017.
- Espay, A. J., et al. "Motor Function in Parkinson's Disease: Evaluation and Management." *Lancet Neurology*, 2021.

Chapter 20. Dermatologic Examination

A. Skin Inspection

1. **Assessing for Color Changes, Lesions, Rashes, or Ulcers**:
   - The skin's color, texture, and appearance offer important diagnostic clues for a variety of systemic and dermatologic conditions. **Color changes** may indicate underlying pathology:
     - **Pallor**: Often seen in **anemia** or **shock**, pallor results from reduced blood flow or decreased red blood cell count. Look for pallor in the mucous membranes, conjunctivae, or nail beds, especially in darker-skinned patients.
     - **Jaundice**: Yellow discoloration of the skin or sclerae suggests **hyperbilirubinemia**, commonly seen in **liver disease** (e.g., cirrhosis, hepatitis) or **hemolysis**.
     - **Cyanosis**: A bluish discoloration of the skin and mucous membranes suggests hypoxia or reduced oxygen saturation. Peripheral cyanosis can occur in **cold environments**, **shock**, or **peripheral vascular disease**, while central cyanosis is typically seen in **cardiac or respiratory disease**.
   - **Lesions** and **rashes** are common findings and can have various causes:
     - **Maculopapular rashes** are often seen in **viral exanthems** (e.g., measles, rubella) or **drug reactions**.
     - **Vesicular lesions** (small, fluid-filled blisters) are typical of **herpes simplex virus** and **varicella-zoster virus** infections.
     - **Ulcers** may be indicative of **diabetes** (neuropathic ulcers), **vascular disease** (arterial or venous ulcers), or **pressure sores**. Assessing the depth, shape, and location of ulcers helps determine the underlying cause.

2. **Differentiating Between Benign and Suspicious Lesions**:
   - The **ABCDE criteria** are commonly used to differentiate between **benign nevi (moles)** and suspicious lesions that may indicate **melanoma**:
     - **A**: **Asymmetry** (melanomas are often asymmetrical, whereas benign lesions are symmetrical).
     - **B**: **Border irregularity** (melanomas tend to have uneven, poorly defined borders).
     - **C**: **Color variation** (melanomas often have multiple colors, including black, brown, red, white, or blue).
     - **D**: **Diameter** greater than 6 mm (though melanomas can be smaller).
     - **E**: **Evolution** or change in size, shape, or color over time.
   - **Seborrheic keratosis** is an example of a benign lesion, appearing as well-defined, raised, and often "stuck on" with a warty surface. **Actinic keratosis**, however, is a precancerous lesion that can progress to **squamous cell carcinoma** and often appears as a rough, scaly patch on sun-exposed areas.

B. Hair and Nails

1. **Observing for Changes in Hair Texture or Distribution**:
   - Changes in **hair texture** or **distribution** can signal systemic or local conditions:
     - **Alopecia**: Hair loss can be patchy or diffuse. **Alopecia areata** is an autoimmune condition leading to patchy hair loss, whereas **androgenic alopecia** (male or female pattern baldness) is due to hormonal factors. **Telogen effluvium** is characterized by diffuse hair thinning triggered by stress, illness, or hormonal changes.
     - **Hirsutism**: Excessive hair growth in women, particularly in a male pattern (e.g., face, chest), suggests **androgen excess**, as seen in conditions like **polycystic ovary syndrome (PCOS)** or **Cushing's syndrome**.
     - **Hair texture**: Dry, brittle hair may suggest **hypothyroidism**, while soft, fine hair may be a sign of **hyperthyroidism**. In addition, **iron deficiency** and **malnutrition** can also lead to changes in hair quality and loss.
2. **Examining Nails for Signs of Systemic Disease (e.g., Clubbing, Splinter Hemorrhages)**:
   - The appearance of the **nails** can provide diagnostic clues for systemic diseases:
     - **Clubbing**: Enlargement of the fingertips and curving of the nails over the fingertips are classic signs of **chronic hypoxia** and are associated with conditions such as **chronic obstructive pulmonary disease (COPD)**, **interstitial lung disease**, and **congenital heart disease**. Clubbing is also seen in **malignancies**, particularly **lung cancer**.
     - **Splinter hemorrhages**: These are small, linear, red-brown streaks under the nails, often associated with **endocarditis**, **vasculitis**, or **trauma**.
     - **Koilonychia** (spoon-shaped nails): This is often seen in **iron deficiency anemia**.
     - **Beau's lines**: Transverse depressions in the nail plate that can indicate **systemic illness**, **chemotherapy**, or **severe malnutrition**.
     - **Onychomycosis**: Fungal infection of the nails presents as **thickened, discolored, or crumbly nails**. This condition is more common in individuals with **diabetes** and **immunosuppression**.

References

- McGee, S. "Evidence-Based Physical Diagnosis." 4th ed., Elsevier, 2017.
- Bickley, L. S. "Bates' Guide to Physical Examination and History Taking." 13th ed., Wolters Kluwer, 2021.
- Elder, D. E., et al. "The ABCDEs of Melanoma." *New England Journal of Medicine*, 2020.

- Olsen, E. A., et al. "Alopecia Areata and Hair Loss: Diagnostic Considerations." *Journal of the American Academy of Dermatology*, 2019.
- de Berker, D., et al. "Nail Disorders and Their Significance in Systemic Disease." *Lancet*, 2018.
- Vora, R. V., et al. "Hair Changes as a Clinical Clue for Systemic Disease." *Indian Dermatology Online Journal*, 2016.
- Rigel, D. S. "Actinic Keratosis and the Risk of Squamous Cell Carcinoma." *Journal of the American Academy of Dermatology*, 2018.

Chapter 21. Genitourinary Examination

A. Male Genitourinary Exam

1. **Inspection and Palpation of the External Genitalia**:
    - The examination of the male external genitalia begins with inspection of the **penis, scrotum**, and **inguinal regions**. Key findings include **lesions, masses, swelling,** or **discoloration**.
        - **Penis**: Inspect the skin for lesions, ulcers, or rashes that may indicate **sexually transmitted infections (STIs)** such as **syphilis** (chancre), **herpes simplex virus (HSV)** (painful vesicles), or **human papillomavirus (HPV)** (genital warts). Inspect the **meatus** for discharge, which may indicate **urethritis** from **gonorrhea** or **chlamydia**.
        - **Scrotum**: Inspect for asymmetry, swelling, or discoloration. **Hydroceles** (fluid around the testicle) can present as a painless scrotal swelling that transilluminates with a light source. **Varicoceles** (enlarged veins in the scrotum) can be palpable as a "bag of worms" and are more common on the left side due to venous drainage patterns.
    - Palpate the **testes** for size, consistency, and tenderness. Normal testes are smooth, firm, and symmetric. **Testicular masses** may indicate **testicular cancer**, which is most common in men aged 15-35. **Epididymitis**, an inflammation of the epididymis, presents as tenderness at the posterior aspect of the testicle, usually due to infection.
    - **Phimosis** (inability to retract the foreskin) or **paraphimosis** (retracted foreskin that cannot be returned) should be noted, as both conditions may require intervention.
2. **Assessing for Hernias, Masses, and Tenderness**:
    - Inspect the **inguinal region** for bulges, which may indicate **inguinal hernias**. Have the patient stand and strain (Valsalva maneuver) to increase intra-abdominal pressure, making hernias more noticeable.
    - **Palpation for hernias**: Palpate the inguinal canal while the patient coughs or strains. A palpable bulge suggests an **inguinal hernia**, which may be reducible (can be pushed back into the abdomen) or non-reducible, raising concern for **incarceration** or **strangulation** .
    - Palpate for **masses** in the testicles and inguinal area, and assess for **tenderness**, which may indicate trauma or infection.

B. Female Genitourinary Exam

1. **Breast Examination Techniques and Identifying Abnormalities**:
    - A **clinical breast examination (CBE)** involves both inspection and palpation to identify potential abnormalities such as **masses, skin changes,** or **nipple discharge**.

- **Inspection**: Have the patient sit with arms at their sides, then raised overhead, and lastly pressing the hands on their hips to tighten the pectoral muscles. Look for **asymmetry**, **skin dimpling**, **retraction of the nipple**, or **erythema**. Skin findings such as **peau d'orange** (orange peel texture) may indicate **breast cancer**.
        - **Palpation**: Using the pads of your fingers, systematically palpate the entire breast, including the **axillary tail** (tail of Spence), in a circular or grid pattern. Palpate for **masses**, noting their size, shape, mobility, and tenderness. A firm, irregular, immobile mass is concerning for **malignancy**, while a smooth, mobile, tender mass suggests a **benign cyst**.
      - Palpate the **axillary lymph nodes** for enlargement, which can occur with **breast cancer**, **mastitis**, or **systemic infections**.
  2. **Examination of the External Genitalia, Including the Vulva, Vagina, and Cervix**:
      - **Vulva**: Inspect for **lesions**, **rashes**, **discharge**, or **erythema**. Lesions such as **genital warts** (HPV), **herpes lesions**, or **syphilitic chancres** should be noted. Palpate for **Bartholin gland cysts** or abscesses, which present as painful swelling near the vaginal opening.
      - **Vagina and cervix**: Insert a lubricated speculum to inspect the vaginal walls and the **cervix**. Assess for **discharge**, which may indicate infection (e.g., **bacterial vaginosis, trichomoniasis, candida**). Inspect the cervix for **erosions**, **ulcers**, or **lesions**, which may suggest **cervical dysplasia** or **cervical cancer**. A **Pap smear** may be performed to screen for cervical cancer, especially in women aged 21-65, as recommended by guidelines.
      - Note any **prolapse** of the pelvic organs, such as **cystocele** or **rectocele**, which may present as a bulge in the vaginal wall.

C. Rectal Examination

  1. **Technique for Assessing Rectal Tone, Prostate in Males, and Checking for Masses or Tenderness**:
      - The **rectal examination** is an important part of both male and female genitourinary assessments, helping to evaluate rectal tone, prostate size, and for the presence of masses.
      - **Assessing rectal tone**: Ask the patient to relax and insert a lubricated, gloved finger into the rectum. **Decreased rectal tone** may indicate **spinal cord injury** or **cauda equina syndrome**, a medical emergency requiring immediate attention.
      - **Prostate examination in males**: Palpate the **prostate gland** through the anterior rectal wall, noting its size, symmetry, consistency, and any nodules or tenderness. A normal prostate feels firm, smooth, and about the size of a walnut. **Prostatitis** may cause the prostate to feel tender, boggy, and enlarged, while

benign prostatic hyperplasia (BPH) presents with a symmetrically enlarged, smooth prostate. **Prostate cancer** may present as hard, irregular nodules.
- **Checking for masses or tenderness**: Palpate the rectum for any **masses**, **polyps**, or **tenderness**. Rectal masses may indicate **colorectal cancer**, especially in older patients. Assess for **hemorrhoids**, **anal fissures**, or **abscesses**, which may present with pain or bleeding.
- In females, the **rectovaginal examination** may help assess the posterior aspect of the uterus and adnexa, as well as rectal integrity, particularly in cases of suspected pelvic masses or **endometriosis**.

References

- McGee, S. "Evidence-Based Physical Diagnosis." 4th ed., Elsevier, 2017.
- Bickley, L. S. "Bates' Guide to Physical Examination and History Taking." 13th ed., Wolters Kluwer, 2021.
- Eisenberg, M. L., & Walsh, T. J. "Male Genital Examination: Diagnostic Clues and Findings." *The Journal of Urology*, 2016.
- American Cancer Society. "Cervical Cancer Screening Guidelines." *ACS Guidelines*, 2021.
- Mohler, J. L., et al. "Prostate Cancer, Version 2.2019, NCCN Clinical Practice Guidelines in Oncology." *Journal of the National Comprehensive Cancer Network*, 2019.
- Goff, B. A., et al. "Pelvic Organ Prolapse: A Review of Diagnostic Techniques and Treatments." *Obstetrics & Gynecology*, 2017.
- Hoffman, B. L., et al. "Williams Gynecology." 4th ed., McGraw Hill, 2020.

Chapter 22. Bedside Diagnostic Techniques

A. Point-of-Care Ultrasound (POCUS)

1. **Integrating Ultrasound for Abdominal, Cardiac, Vascular, and Thoracic Assessments**:
    - **Point-of-Care Ultrasound (POCUS)** has revolutionized bedside diagnostics, offering real-time imaging that aids in rapid diagnosis and decision-making. POCUS is increasingly used in emergency and critical care settings for a variety of **abdominal, cardiac, vascular**, and **thoracic assessments**.
    - **Abdominal assessment**: POCUS is highly effective in evaluating **free fluid** (e.g., **ascites, hemoperitoneum**), and identifying **abdominal aortic aneurysms (AAA)**. The **FAST (Focused Assessment with Sonography for Trauma)** exam is a specific protocol to detect free intraperitoneal or pericardial fluid in trauma patients .
    - **Cardiac assessment**: POCUS allows for the rapid evaluation of **left ventricular function, pericardial effusion**, and **volume status** by assessing the **inferior vena cava (IVC)**. It is particularly useful in the evaluation of **undifferentiated shock, acute heart failure**, or **cardiac tamponade**. Studies have shown that focused cardiac ultrasound can reduce time to diagnosis in critically ill patients .
    - **Vascular assessment**: **Ultrasound-guided vascular access** is the gold standard for placing central lines, minimizing complications such as pneumothorax. Additionally, POCUS is used to assess for **deep vein thrombosis (DVT)** by compressing the veins in the lower extremities to check for thrombus .
    - **Thoracic assessment**: POCUS is critical for detecting **pleural effusions, pneumothorax, pulmonary edema**, and **pneumonia**. **Lung ultrasound** is more sensitive than chest X-ray for detecting pleural effusions and pneumothorax, providing quick, bedside visualization of lung sliding and pleural line abnormalities. The **B-line** artifact in lung ultrasound indicates **interstitial syndrome**, often seen in **pulmonary edema** or **ARDS** .
2. **Key advantages of POCUS** include its **non-invasive, real-time** nature, and its capacity to provide immediate diagnostic information without radiation exposure. Studies have demonstrated that POCUS improves diagnostic accuracy and reduces time to intervention in emergency and critical care settings .

B. EKG (ECG) Interpretation

1. **Basics of ECG Interpretation During Physical Exams**:
    - **Electrocardiogram (ECG)** is a fundamental bedside diagnostic tool for assessing **cardiac rhythm, conduction abnormalities**, and **ischemic changes**. Correct interpretation of ECG findings can assist in the rapid diagnosis

of **acute coronary syndromes, arrhythmias, electrolyte imbalances**, and other cardiac pathologies.
- **Rate and rhythm**: Calculate the heart rate by measuring the RR interval (300 divided by the number of large boxes between QRS complexes). Assess the rhythm for **regularity** or **irregularity**, which helps diagnose conditions like **atrial fibrillation** (irregularly irregular rhythm), **ventricular tachycardia**, or **bradyarrhythmias**.
- **P wave and PR interval**: Analyze the **P waves** for shape and consistency to diagnose **atrial hypertrophy** or **atrial enlargement**. The **PR interval** reflects atrioventricular conduction, and **prolonged PR intervals** indicate **first-degree heart block**.
- **QRS complex**: Assess the **QRS duration** for ventricular conduction abnormalities. A **widened QRS** suggests **bundle branch block** or **ventricular tachycardia**. Examine for **pathologic Q waves** that signify prior **myocardial infarction (MI)**.
- **ST segment and T wave**: Look for **ST-segment elevation** (seen in **STEMI**) or **depression** (indicative of ischemia). **T-wave inversion** can be seen in **ischemia, electrolyte imbalances**, or **pericarditis**.
- **QT interval**: Prolonged **QT interval** increases the risk of **torsades de pointes** and can be caused by medications, electrolyte disturbances, or congenital syndromes.
2. Rapid ECG interpretation during a physical exam is critical for diagnosing **acute myocardial infarction, atrial fibrillation**, and **other life-threatening arrhythmias**. Studies have shown that timely interpretation of ECGs, particularly in the context of acute chest pain, significantly improves patient outcomes.

C. Pulmonary Function Testing (PFTs)

1. **Using Spirometry at the Bedside for Initial Evaluation**:
    - **Spirometry** is a key diagnostic tool for assessing **lung function** at the bedside, particularly in patients with **asthma, chronic obstructive pulmonary disease (COPD)**, or other obstructive and restrictive lung diseases. It measures the volume of air the patient can exhale and the speed of the exhalation, providing critical information about airflow limitation.
    - **Forced Vital Capacity (FVC)**: This is the total amount of air that the patient can forcibly exhale after taking a deep breath. A **reduced FVC** suggests **restrictive lung disease**, where lung expansion is impaired due to conditions like **pulmonary fibrosis** or **pleural effusion**.
    - **Forced Expiratory Volume in 1 second (FEV1)**: This is the volume of air exhaled during the first second of the FVC maneuver. A reduced FEV1, particularly with a low FEV1/FVC ratio, is indicative of **obstructive lung disease**, such as **asthma** or **COPD**.

- **FEV1/FVC ratio**: This ratio helps differentiate between obstructive and restrictive lung diseases. A ratio of less than 0.70 is typical of obstructive lung disease, while a normal or high ratio with reduced FVC suggests restrictive disease.
- Spirometry is a **non-invasive**, quick, and highly effective tool for evaluating respiratory function at the bedside. In patients with **acute exacerbations of asthma** or **COPD**, bedside spirometry can aid in assessing the severity of airflow obstruction and guide treatment decisions.

2. The use of bedside **spirometry** has been shown to improve **asthma management** in acute care settings and is valuable in the **early detection** of respiratory compromise in patients with **COPD**, leading to better long-term outcomes.

References

- McGee, S. "Evidence-Based Physical Diagnosis." 4th ed., Elsevier, 2017.
- Bickley, L. S. "Bates' Guide to Physical Examination and History Taking." 13th ed., Wolters Kluwer, 2021.
- Moore, C. L., et al. "Point-of-Care Ultrasound in Emergency and Critical Care Medicine." *New England Journal of Medicine*, 2019.
- Spencer, K. T., et al. "Focused Cardiac Ultrasound: A Fundamental Tool for the Modern Cardiologist." *Journal of the American Society of Echocardiography*, 2018.
- Nazerian, P., et al. "Lung Ultrasound for the Diagnosis of Pneumonia in the Emergency Department: A Meta-analysis." *European Journal of Emergency Medicine*, 2019.
- Volpicelli, G., et al. "International Evidence-Based Recommendations for Point-of-Care Lung Ultrasound." *Intensive Care Medicine*, 2017.
- Nishimura, R. A., et al. "2017 AHA/ACC Focused Update of the 2014 AHA/ACC Guideline for the Management of Patients with Valvular Heart Disease." *Journal of the American College of Cardiology*, 2017.
- Thygesen, K., et al. "Fourth Universal Definition of Myocardial Infarction." *European Heart Journal*, 2018.
- Pellegrino, R., et al. "Interpretative Strategies for Lung Function Tests." *European Respiratory Journal*, 2019.
- Global Initiative for Chronic Obstructive Lung Disease (GOLD). "Global Strategy for the Diagnosis, Management, and Prevention of COPD." *GOLD Report*, 2021.

Chapter 23. Special Considerations in the Physical Exam

A. Elderly Patients

1. **Adjustments for Frail or Elderly Patients with Mobility Issues**:
    - The physical examination of elderly patients often requires modifications due to **mobility issues**, **frailty**, and the presence of multiple **comorbidities**. **Aging** affects nearly every system of the body, and clinicians must be mindful of these changes to avoid discomfort or harm.
    - **Positioning and Mobility**: Many elderly patients may have limited mobility due to **arthritis**, **osteoporosis**, or previous injuries (e.g., hip fractures). These conditions can make certain exam maneuvers difficult or painful. It's essential to position patients comfortably and adjust the exam accordingly. For instance, instead of having the patient lie flat for an abdominal exam, use a slight head elevation to avoid discomfort due to **kyphosis** (forward curving of the spine common in the elderly).
    - **Balance and Gait Assessment**: Gait assessment is critical in elderly patients to evaluate the risk of falls. The **Timed Up and Go (TUG) test** is a validated tool for assessing mobility and fall risk in older adults. Patients are asked to rise from a chair, walk 3 meters, turn, walk back, and sit down. A time of more than 12 seconds indicates an increased risk of falls.
    - **Skin Integrity and Pressure Ulcers**: Elderly patients, especially those who are bedridden or immobile, are at increased risk for **pressure ulcers**. These can develop quickly and should be examined closely, particularly over bony prominences. Inspection for **bruising**, **skin tears**, or **pressure injuries** is crucial, as the elderly often have thinner, more fragile skin.
    - **Hearing and Vision**: It's important to check for **hearing impairment** (common in up to 60% of adults over age 70) and **visual deficits**. Speaking clearly and at an appropriate volume, as well as ensuring proper lighting for visual tasks, improves communication and patient cooperation.

B. Obese Patients

1. **Overcoming Challenges in Examining Obese Patients**:
    - Obese patients present unique challenges during the physical exam due to increased body mass and potential comorbidities like **diabetes**, **hypertension**, and **obstructive sleep apnea** (OSA). Adjustments in technique and equipment are necessary for an accurate and comfortable examination.
    - **Proper Equipment**: Use appropriately sized **blood pressure cuffs**, as using a cuff that is too small can lead to falsely elevated readings. The cuff should encircle **80% of the arm circumference**. Larger patients may require **bariatric exam tables** and **chairs** with proper weight limits to ensure safety and comfort.

- **Palpation and Auscultation**: Palpating through **thick subcutaneous fat** can make it more difficult to assess for **masses**, **organomegaly**, or **pulses**. When palpating the abdomen, it may be necessary to apply deeper pressure to feel structures such as the liver, spleen, and kidneys. For **auscultation**, especially of the heart and lungs, consider having the patient sit forward or adjust their position to help shift adipose tissue for clearer auscultation.
- **Cardiopulmonary Exam**: In obese patients, **obstructive sleep apnea (OSA)** and **heart failure** are common comorbidities, which necessitate careful attention to cardiopulmonary function. **Jugular venous pressure (JVP)** may be difficult to assess due to a short, thick neck, and **hepatomegaly** can be challenging to palpate. Use ultrasound as an adjunct to detect conditions like **heart failure** or **hepatic congestion**.
- **Skin Folds**: Obese patients are at increased risk for **intertrigo** (inflammation in skin folds), **fungal infections**, and **pressure ulcers**. Carefully inspect **skin folds**, such as the **axilla**, **inguinal folds**, and **submammary areas**, for **erythema**, **moisture**, and **infections** like **candidiasis**.

C. Pediatric Examination

1. **Special Approaches for Pediatric Patients**:
   - Performing physical exams in children requires a patient, flexible approach that adapts to the child's **developmental stage** and **comfort level**. Pediatric patients, especially infants and toddlers, may not cooperate fully, so the sequence of the exam often needs to be adjusted.
   - **Infants and Toddlers**: The examination of infants should start with **observation** and **non-invasive procedures** such as auscultation, which can be done while the child is calm or held by a caregiver. Save invasive or uncomfortable procedures (e.g., **otoscopic exam**, **throat inspection**) for last. During the exam, monitor for **developmental milestones** such as head control, crawling, or standing to assess the child's overall growth and development.
   - **Engaging School-Age Children**: School-age children can often follow directions, so explaining the steps of the exam in simple terms can reduce anxiety. Use distraction techniques, such as involving the child in the process (e.g., letting them hold the stethoscope), or engaging in conversation to help them relax.
   - **Assessing Growth**: In pediatric exams, **growth charts** are essential for tracking **height**, **weight**, and **head circumference**. Regular use of these charts helps monitor for **failure to thrive**, **obesity**, or **delayed growth**. In adolescence, **puberty staging** (Tanner staging) is critical for assessing normal development.
   - **Cardiac Exam**: Pediatric patients can have **innocent murmurs**, but a thorough auscultation should assess for any concerning findings such as **harsh murmurs**, **wide pulse pressure**, or **failure to thrive**, which could indicate congenital heart

defects. **Peripheral pulses** should be checked to rule out **coarctation of the aorta**.
- **Neurological Exam**: The neurological exam in infants includes assessing **reflexes** such as the **Moro reflex** and **Babinski reflex**. In older children, testing **balance**, **coordination**, and **fine motor skills** becomes important, as developmental delays can become more evident .
- **Parental Involvement**: Involving the parents during the examination provides comfort to the child and can improve cooperation. Educating parents on developmental milestones and anticipatory guidance regarding safety, nutrition, and immunizations is a critical part of pediatric care.

References

- Bickley, L. S. "Bates' Guide to Physical Examination and History Taking." 13th ed., Wolters Kluwer, 2021.
- McGee, S. "Evidence-Based Physical Diagnosis." 4th ed., Elsevier, 2017.
- American Geriatrics Society. "Guidelines for the Care of Older Adults." *Journal of the American Geriatrics Society*, 2021.
- Guralnik, J. M., et al. "The Timed Up and Go Test: Predicting Falls in Older Adults." *Journal of the American Geriatrics Society*, 2020.
- Jensen, M. D., et al. "Obesity in Adults: Etiology and Treatment." *Journal of the American Medical Association*, 2019.
- Ogden, C. L., et al. "Growth Charts for Children with Special Health Care Needs." *Pediatrics*, 2020.
- American Academy of Pediatrics. "Bright Futures Guidelines for Health Supervision of Infants, Children, and Adolescents." 4th ed., 2017.

Chapter 24. Common Physical Exam Findings and Clinical Correlations at Wynn Medical Center

The physical exam remains a vital diagnostic tool in internal medicine, offering immediate clues to disease processes. Through case-based learning, we can illustrate how common physical exam findings correlate with underlying pathologies and inform the diagnostic work-up.

A. Case-Based Learning

Heart Failure

A 65-year-old Vietnamese male presents with **dyspnea on exertion**, **orthopnea**, and **lower extremity swelling**. He has a history of **hypertension** and **coronary artery disease**.
Physical Exam Findings:

- **Jugular Venous Distension (JVD)**: Elevated **jugular venous pressure** suggests increased right atrial pressure, commonly seen in **right-sided heart failure** or **biventricular failure**. JVD correlates with increased **central venous pressure** and fluid overload.
- **Bibasilar crackles**: Fine crackles in both lung bases are a sign of **pulmonary edema** due to **left-sided heart failure**. The presence of pulmonary congestion reflects fluid accumulation in the alveoli, impairing gas exchange.
- **Pitting edema**: Bilateral lower extremity edema is commonly seen in **congestive heart failure** (CHF) and results from **venous congestion** due to increased systemic venous pressure.
- **S3 gallop**: The presence of an **S3** heart sound is a hallmark of **volume overload** and can be heard in systolic heart failure. It is caused by rapid filling of a dilated ventricle during early diastole.

2. **Clinical Implications**: These findings suggest **congestive heart failure**, likely secondary to the patient's history of **coronary artery disease** and **hypertension**. The physical exam findings guide the initial work-up:
    - **Diagnostic Work-up**: **Echocardiogram** to assess **left ventricular function** (ejection fraction), chest X-ray to evaluate for **pulmonary edema**, and **BNP (B-type natriuretic peptide)** to gauge heart failure severity. Elevated BNP correlates with increased ventricular filling pressures.

Cirrhosis

A 52-year-old Chinese male with a history of **alcohol abuse** presents with **abdominal distention** and **jaundice**.
Physical Exam Findings:

- **Jaundice**: Yellow discoloration of the skin and sclera indicates **hyperbilirubinemia**, often due to **hepatic dysfunction**. In cirrhosis, the liver's ability to conjugate and excrete bilirubin is impaired, leading to its accumulation.
- **Ascites**: Fluid accumulation in the abdominal cavity, causing **abdominal distention**, is a hallmark of **portal hypertension** secondary to cirrhosis. **Shifting dullness** and the **fluid wave test** help confirm ascites.
- **Palmar erythema** and **spider angiomas**: These findings are seen in **chronic liver disease** and are related to increased levels of circulating estrogens due to impaired liver metabolism.
- **Asterixis**: A flapping tremor observed when the patient extends their hands, indicative of **hepatic encephalopathy**. This results from the accumulation of ammonia and other toxins due to liver dysfunction.

3. **Clinical Implications**: The findings suggest **advanced cirrhosis**, likely due to chronic alcohol use, with complications of **portal hypertension** and **hepatic encephalopathy**. Immediate diagnostic steps include:
    - **Diagnostic Work-up**: **Abdominal ultrasound** to assess liver size, texture, and the presence of ascites. **Liver function tests (LFTs)** to assess hepatic injury, **serum albumin** and **coagulation studies** for liver synthetic function, and **ammonia levels** to evaluate for hepatic encephalopathy. **Paracentesis** may be performed to assess ascitic fluid for infection (spontaneous bacterial peritonitis).

Pneumonia

A 45-year-old Hispanic woman presents with a **productive cough**, **fever**, and **shortness of breath** for 3 days.
Physical Exam Findings:

- **Fever**: An elevated temperature is commonly associated with **bacterial infections**, such as pneumonia.
- **Crackles**: Fine or coarse crackles (rales) heard over a lung field suggest **alveolar filling**, which is typical of **lobar pneumonia**. The crackles occur due to fluid, pus, or inflammation within the alveoli.
- **Increased tactile fremitus** and **dullness to percussion**: These findings occur over areas of lung consolidation. In pneumonia, alveoli fill with exudate, which conducts sound and vibration more effectively than air, causing increased fremitus and dullness.
- **Egophony**: When auscultating, if the patient's voice sounds like "A" when saying "E," it suggests **lung consolidation**, a characteristic finding in pneumonia.

4. **Clinical Implications**: The classic signs point to **community-acquired pneumonia**, likely bacterial in origin. The combination of **fever**, **productive cough**, and **focal crackles** increases the likelihood of this diagnosis. A targeted work-up would include:

- **Diagnostic Work-up**: **Chest X-ray** to confirm the presence of consolidation and **sputum cultures** to identify the causative organism. Blood cultures may be considered in patients with severe pneumonia or suspected bacteremia. The **CURB-65 score** can help assess the severity and guide management (whether outpatient or inpatient treatment).

Eczema (Atopic Dermatitis)

Case Example:
A 28-year-old female presents with **itchy**, **dry patches** of skin on her arms and behind her knees. She reports a history of **seasonal allergies** and **asthma**.

Physical Exam Findings:

- **Dry, scaly patches**: Typically found on the **flexural surfaces** (e.g., elbows, behind the knees), indicative of **chronic atopic dermatitis**. The skin may appear **lichenified** due to chronic scratching.
- **Erythematous, excoriated lesions**: Red, inflamed skin with scratch marks is common in active flare-ups of **eczema**.
- **Xerosis (dry skin)**: Generalized **dryness** of the skin is a hallmark of **atopic dermatitis**.
- **Dennie-Morgan lines**: Prominent folds or lines under the lower eyelids, often associated with **atopy**.

Clinical Implications: Eczema, particularly in a patient with a history of **atopy** (asthma and allergies), is part of the **atopic triad**. Chronic inflammation and barrier dysfunction lead to **dry, itchy skin** and **secondary infections** from scratching. Managing the condition requires controlling both **inflammation** and **dryness**.

Diagnostic Work-up:

- Typically, **eczema** is diagnosed **clinically** based on the pattern of skin involvement and history of atopy. No specific laboratory tests are required unless secondary bacterial infection is suspected, in which case a **skin culture** may be taken. Treatment typically involves **topical corticosteroids, moisturizers**, and **antihistamines** to control itching.

Chronic Obstructive Pulmonary Disease (COPD)

A 64-year-old Vietnamese male with a 40-year history of smoking presents with **shortness of breath** and **chronic cough**, producing **white sputum**.

Physical Exam Findings:

- **Barrel chest**: Increased **anteroposterior diameter** of the chest is a classic finding in patients with **COPD**, reflecting **chronic lung hyperinflation**.
- **Prolonged expiratory phase**: This occurs due to airflow obstruction, a hallmark of COPD. Wheezing and decreased breath sounds are common.
- **Pursed-lip breathing**: Patients with COPD often use this technique to maintain positive pressure in the airways and improve oxygenation.
- **Clubbing**: While not common in COPD, it can be seen if **hypoxemia** is severe or if **lung cancer** is a comorbidity.
- **Use of accessory muscles**: During respiration, especially in advanced COPD, patients may visibly use **sternocleidomastoid and intercostal muscles** to help breathe due to increased work of breathing.

Clinical Implications: COPD is characterized by **chronic airway obstruction**, often due to **emphysema** or **chronic bronchitis**, primarily caused by smoking. The patient's **barrel chest**, **wheezing**, and prolonged expiratory phase indicate **severe airflow limitation** and **hyperinflation** of the lungs.

Diagnostic Work-up:

- **Pulmonary Function Tests (PFTs)**: A **spirometry** showing a **reduced FEV1/FVC ratio** (<0.70) confirms **obstructive lung disease**.
- **Chest X-ray**: To assess for **hyperinflation**, flattened diaphragms, and possible complications like **bullae**.
- **Arterial Blood Gas (ABG)**: In cases of severe disease or respiratory failure, an ABG can show **hypoxemia** or **hypercapnia**.
- **Alpha-1 Antitrypsin Levels**: Consider in younger patients or non-smokers with COPD to rule out a genetic cause.

Type 2 Diabetes Mellitus

A 55-year-old Caucasian female with a history of **hypertension** and a **BMI of 32** presents with **increased thirst, frequent urination**, and **fatigue**.

Physical Exam Findings:

- **Acanthosis nigricans**: Dark, velvety patches on the back of the neck and in skin folds, often associated with **insulin resistance**.
- **Obesity**: Central adiposity is commonly seen in patients with type 2 diabetes, reflecting **metabolic syndrome**.
- **Decreased sensation in the feet**: Diabetic **peripheral neuropathy** is common, particularly in long-standing or poorly controlled diabetes.

- **Non-healing ulcers**: Patients with **diabetic neuropathy** and **poor circulation** may develop ulcers, particularly on the feet, that are slow to heal.

Clinical Implications: Type 2 diabetes is characterized by **insulin resistance**, and obesity is a key risk factor. Physical exam findings such as **acanthosis nigricans** and **peripheral neuropathy** are indicative of **long-standing hyperglycemia** and potential complications. Early diagnosis and control of blood sugar levels can prevent progression to more severe complications like **diabetic foot ulcers** or **nephropathy**.

Diagnostic Work-up:

- **Fasting plasma glucose (FPG)** or **HbA1c**: FPG ≥ 126 mg/dL or HbA1c ≥ 6.5% confirms **type 2 diabetes**.
- **Oral glucose tolerance test (OGTT)**: Can be used to diagnose prediabetes and diabetes in uncertain cases.
- **Urine microalbumin**: To assess for early signs of **diabetic nephropathy**.
- **Lipid profile**: Dyslipidemia is common in diabetic patients and increases the risk for **cardiovascular disease**.

Urinary Tract Infection (UTI)

Case Example:
A 32-year-old female presents with **dysuria**, **increased urinary frequency**, and **suprapubic discomfort** for the past 2 days. She denies fever or flank pain.

Physical Exam Findings:

- **Suprapubic tenderness**: Mild tenderness over the bladder may be present in cases of **acute cystitis**.
- **Absence of costovertebral angle (CVA) tenderness**: Differentiates **uncomplicated UTI** (cystitis) from **pyelonephritis** (kidney infection). In pyelonephritis, there would be significant **CVA tenderness** and possibly fever.
- **Normal vital signs**: The absence of fever, hypotension, or tachycardia suggests the UTI is confined to the bladder and not causing systemic infection (sepsis).

Clinical Implications: This patient has the typical presentation of **acute uncomplicated cystitis**, a lower urinary tract infection common in young women. Physical findings, such as suprapubic tenderness without fever or CVA tenderness, point to a localized infection rather than a more severe complication like **pyelonephritis**.

Diagnostic Work-up:

- **Urinalysis**: Look for **pyuria** (white blood cells), **bacteriuria**, **nitrites**, and **leukocyte esterase**, which are typical in UTIs.
- **Urine culture**: To identify the causative organism, especially in recurrent UTIs or cases where initial treatment fails.
- **Pregnancy test**: Recommended for women of childbearing age to rule out pregnancy as a cause of urinary symptoms, which can mimic UTI.

B. Integrating Physical Exam Findings with Diagnostic Work-Up

The physical examination not only provides immediate diagnostic clues but also directs the subsequent diagnostic work-up. Here are ways to integrate physical exam findings into the broader clinical context:

- **Diagnostic imaging**: Physical exam findings such as **rales**, **wheezing**, or **asymmetric lung sounds** often lead to **chest X-rays** or **CT scans** for further evaluation. For example, a patient with **dullness to percussion** and **absent breath sounds** may have a **pleural effusion**, which can be confirmed and quantified by **thoracic ultrasound** or **chest X-ray**.
- **Laboratory tests**: In the setting of **pallor** and **tachycardia**, physical exam findings may suggest **anemia**, prompting a **complete blood count (CBC)** to assess hemoglobin levels. Likewise, **elevated JVP** and **pitting edema** may lead to ordering **BNP levels** to evaluate for heart failure.
- **Bedside procedures**: For a patient with ascites on physical exam (e.g., **shifting dullness**), a **diagnostic paracentesis** would be performed to assess the cause (e.g., cirrhosis vs. malignancy vs. heart failure).

Chapter 25. Putting All Together: Master the History Taking Skills and Physical Exam at Wynn Medical Center

1. **Essential Skills for the Residents**:
    - **Comprehensive taking history and physical examination skills** are foundational for internal medicine residents, forming the basis for accurate diagnosis, management, and patient care. Mastering these skills requires a detailed understanding of both normal and abnormal findings and the ability to correlate them with underlying pathologies.
    - **Observation and inspection** are critical first steps in any physical examination, whether assessing a patient's general appearance, skin integrity, or respiratory effort. Subtle visual clues such as **jaundice**, **clubbing**, or **postural changes** can provide early indications of systemic disease.
    - **Palpation** plays a crucial role in detecting organ enlargement, masses, or tenderness. For example, detecting **hepatosplenomegaly** through abdominal palpation can lead to early identification of hematologic conditions or cirrhosis, while palpating for **tenderness** over joints or bones can point toward musculoskeletal or systemic inflammatory diseases.
    - **Auscultation** allows for the detection of crucial cardiovascular, pulmonary, and abdominal abnormalities. Identifying abnormal heart sounds like **murmurs** or **gallops**, detecting **crackles** in the lungs, or listening for **bruits** over arteries can help diagnose heart failure, pneumonia, or vascular occlusions.
    - **Neurological and musculoskeletal exams** provide vital insights into patient function, especially for detecting deficits such as **weakness**, **sensory loss**, **reflex changes**, and **coordination difficulties**. These findings guide further testing, imaging, and management decisions.
2. **Encouraging Continued Practice and Refinement of History Taking and Examination Techniques**:
    - **Continual refinement of physical examination skills** is essential as internal medicine residents progress through their training. The learning process should involve frequent **hands-on practice** with diverse patient populations, as well as **mentorship** from experienced clinicians who can provide valuable feedback on technique.
    - **Critical thinking** and **clinical reasoning** should be integrated with physical exam findings. Residents must constantly ask themselves, "What does this finding mean?" and "How does this influence my differential diagnosis?" This approach encourages not only the honing of physical skills but also the development of the resident's clinical acumen.
    - Residents should be encouraged to adopt a **systematic approach** to the exam—ensuring no system is overlooked—and to adapt their methods to accommodate different patient populations, including the elderly, pediatric, and obese patients. As emphasized throughout the training, a thorough physical exam is integral to detecting signs that laboratory tests or imaging may not reveal.

- **Bedside diagnostic tools** like **point-of-care ultrasound (POCUS)** and **spirometry** are becoming increasingly integrated into physical examination, offering additional real-time insights that can sharpen diagnostic accuracy. Familiarity with these technologies, alongside traditional examination techniques, enhances diagnostic capability.
- **Continued self-assessment** through case reviews, simulations, and patient outcomes is crucial. Residents should revisit cases where physical exam findings significantly contributed to diagnosis or where they may have been missed. Reflecting on these cases strengthens their skills for future encounters.
- Lastly, **lifelong learning** is essential in internal medicine. Advances in diagnostic technology, disease understanding, and patient care approaches will continue to evolve, and residents must stay current with **best practices** while maintaining a commitment to **mastery of the physical exam**.

Part 3: Blood Labs and EKG Interpretations

Chapter 26. Common Blood Tests

A. Complete Blood Count

> *A Complete Blood Count (CBC) is a blood test that provides information about the types and numbers of blood cells in the body, including red blood cells, white blood cells, and platelets.*
>
> *It helps diagnose conditions such as anemia, infection, other blood disorders and also monitors overall health and response to treatment.*
>
> *This test measures parameters like hemoglobin, white blood cell count, and platelet count, providing valuable insights into the patient's health status.*

Test	Description	Normal Range
Hemoglobin (Hb)	Amount of oxygen-carrying protein in the blood	• Adult male: 13.8 - 17.2 g/dL • Adult female: 12.1 - 15.1 g/dL
Hematocrit (Hct)	Percentage of blood volume occupied by red blood cells	• Adult male: 40.7% - 50.3% • Adult female: 36.1% - 44.3%
Red Blood Cell (RBC)	Number of red blood cells per volume of blood	• Adult male: 4.7 - 6.1 cells/mcL • Adult female: 4.2 - 5.4 cells/mcL
Mean Corpuscular Volume (MCV)	Average volume of red blood cells	80 - 100 fL
Mean Corpuscular Hemoglobin (MCH)	Average amount of hemoglobin per red blood cell	27 - 33 pg
Mean Corpuscular Hemoglobin Concentration (MCHC)	Concentration of hemoglobin in red blood cells	32% - 36%
Red Cell Distribution Width (RDW)	Variation in red blood cell size	11.5% - 14.5 %
White Blood Cell Count (WBC)	Number of white blood cells per volume of blood	4,500 - 11,000 cells/mcL
Platelet Count	Number of platelets per volume of blood	150,000 - 400,000 cells/mcL

Interpretation

- Abnormalities in the CBC may indicate various conditions such as anemia, infection, inflammation, or bleeding disorders.
- High or low values should be interpreted in clinical context, other lab findings and patient history to determine the underlying cause and appropriate management.

- Hemoglobin (Hb), Hematocrit (Hct), White Blood Cell Count (WBC), Platelet Count: Assess for anemia, infection, inflammation, and thrombocytopenia or thrombocytosis.

B. Comprehensive Metabolic Panel

> ➤ *The Comprehensive Metabolic Panel (CMP) is a blood test that assesses various aspects of a person's metabolism and organ function.*
>
> ➤ *It includes measurements of glucose, electrolytes, kidney function, liver function, and protein levels.*
>
> ➤ *The CMP helps diagnose conditions such as diabetes, kidney disease, and liver disorders, and monitors overall health and response to treatment.*

Test		Description	Normal Range
Glucose		Blood sugar levels	70 - 100 mg/dL (when fasting)
Blood Urea Nitrogen (BUN)		Amount of nitrogen in blood coming from urea	7 - 20 mg/dL
Creatinine		Amount of creatinine in blood to measure kidney function	• Male: 0.6 - 1.3 mg/dL • Female: 0.5 - 1.1 mg/dL
Electro-lytes	Sodium (Na)	Maintains proper balance of water and minerals, an important role in nerve and muscle function	80 - 100 fL
	Potassium (K)	Important for nerve function and muscle contractions	2.5 - 5.0 mEq/L
	Chloride (Cl)	Maintains fluid balance	98 - 106 mEg/L
	Carbon Dioxide (CO2)	Reflects the body's acid-base balance	22- 29 mEq/L
Total Protein		Amount of protein in the blood	6.0 - 8.3 g/dL
Albumin		A type of protein made by the liver to help maintain blood volume and pressure	3.5 - 5.0 g/dL
Total Bilirubin		Amount of bilirubin in the blood. An elevated level indicates liver or bile duct dysfunction	0.1 - 1.2 mg/dL
Alkaline Phosphatase (ALP)		An enzyme found in various tissues, mainly in the liver and bones. Elevated level indicates liver or bone disease	44 - 147 IU/L
Alanine Aminotransferase		Enzymes found in the liver. Elevated level indicates	• ALT: 7 - 56 IU/L

(ALT) and Aspartate Aminotransferase (AST)	liver damage	• AST: 10 - 40 IU/L

Interpretation
- Abnormalities in the CMP may indicate various conditions such as kidney or liver disease, electrolyte imbalances, or acid-base disorders.
- High or low values should be interpreted in a clinical context, other lab findings, and patient history to determine the underlying cause and appropriate management.

C. Urinalysis

> ➢ *Urinalysis (UA) is a common diagnostic test that examines the physical, chemical, and microscopic properties of urine.*
> ➢ *It assesses hydration status, kidney function, and detects conditions like urinary tract infections, kidney stones, or diabetes.*
> ➢ *The test involves analyzing urine for color, clarity, pH, protein, glucose, blood cells, and bacteria under a microscope.*

Physical Appearance Observation
- Color: Normal urine color ranges from pale yellow to amber. Abnormal colors may indicate various conditions such as dehydration, liver disease, or urinary tract infections.
- Clarity: Normal urine is clear. Cloudy urine may indicate the presence of bacteria, pus, or other substances.

Chemical Examination

Examination	Description	Interpretation
pH	Measures the acidity or alkalinity of urine	• Normal range: 4.6 to 8.0 • Abnormal specific gravity may indicate dehydration, kidney dysfunction, or diabetes
Specific Gravity	Measures urine concentration	• Normal range: 1.005 to 1.030 • Abnormal specific gravity may indicate dehydration, kidney dysfunction, or diabetes

Protein	Detects the presence of protein in urine	Abnormal levels may indicate kidney disease such as diabetic kidney disease, multiple myeloma, or problems in pregnancy
Glucose	Detects the presence of glucose in urine	Abnormal levels may indicate diabetes or kidney dysfunction
Ketones	Detects the presence of ketones in urine	Abnormal levels may indicate diabetic ketoacidosis, starvation, or certain metabolic disorders
Blood	Detects the presence of red blood cells in urine	Abnormal levels may indicate urinary tract infections or malignancy, kidney stones, kidney cysts or other kidney conditions
Nitrites	Detects the presence of bacteria that convert nitrate to nitrite in urine	Abnormal levels may indicate urinary tract infections

Microscopic Examination

- Red Blood Cells (RBCs): Normal range: **0-2 RBCs per high-power field (HPF).** Elevated levels may indicate kidney disease, urinary tract infections, or other conditions.
- White Blood Cells (WBCs): Normal range: **0-5 WBCs per HPF.** Elevated levels may indicate urinary tract infections or inflammation.
- Bacteria: The presence of bacteria in urine may indicate urinary tract infections.
- Crystals: The presence of crystals in urine may indicate kidney stones or metabolic disorders.

Interpretation

- Abnormalities in urinalysis results may indicate various urinary tract disorders, kidney dysfunction, metabolic disorders, or systemic diseases.
- Results should be interpreted in conjunction with other clinical findings and patient history to determine the underlying cause and appropriate management.

D. Lipid Panel

> - *A lipid panel is a blood test that measures levels of cholesterol and triglycerides, essential for assessing cardiovascular health and risk factors.*
> - *It typically includes measurements of total cholesterol, HDL cholesterol (good cholesterol), LDL cholesterol (bad cholesterol), and triglycerides.*
> - *The results can guide the APh in managing cholesterol levels to reduce the risk of heart disease and stroke.*

Type	Description	Range
Total Cholesterol	Desirable	<200 mg/dL
	Borderline high	200-239 mg/dL
	High	240 mg/dL and above
Low-density Lipoprotein (LDL) Cholesterol	Optimal	<100 mg/dL
	Near optimal/above optimal	100-129 mg/dL
	Borderline high	130-159 mg/dL
	High	160-189 mg/dL
	Very high	190 mg/dL and above
High-density Lipoprotein (HDL) Cholesterol	Low (increased risk)	• <40 mg/dL (men) • <50 mg/dL (women)
	Good	• 40-59 mg/dL (men) • 50-59 mg/dL (women)
	High (protective)	60 mg/dL and above
Triglycerides	Normal	<150 mg/dL

Type	Description	Range
	Borderline high	150-199 mg/dL
	High	200-499 mg/dL
	Very high	500 mg/dL and above
Non-HDL Cholesterol	Goal	30 mg/dL higher than the LDL cholesterol level

Interpretation

- High levels of total cholesterol, LDL cholesterol, and triglycerides, as well as low levels of HDL cholesterol, are associated with an increased risk of cardiovascular disease.
- Elevated LDL cholesterol is particularly concerning as it can lead to the buildup of plaque in the arteries, increasing the risk of heart disease and stroke.
- Low HDL cholesterol is also a risk factor for cardiovascular disease, as HDL helps remove LDL cholesterol from the bloodstream.
- Triglyceride levels may be influenced by factors such as diet, physical activity, and alcohol consumption. Elevated triglyceride levels are associated with an increased risk of heart disease, especially when combined with other lipid abnormalities.

In addition to lipid levels, other factors such as age, gender, blood pressure, smoking status, diabetes, and family history of cardiovascular disease should be considered when assessing overall cardiovascular risk.

E. Thyroid Panel

> ➢ A thyroid panel is a blood test that assesses thyroid function by measuring levels of thyroid hormones and thyroid-stimulating hormone (TSH).
>
> ➢ It helps diagnose thyroid disorders such as hypothyroidism, hyperthyroidism, and autoimmune thyroid diseases.
>
> ➢ The panel typically includes measurements of TSH, free thyroxine (T4), and sometimes triiodothyronine (T3) levels.

Type	Description	Range
Thyroid-Stimulating Hormone (TSH)	Normal range	Typically between 0.4 to 4.0 mIU/L
	Elevated TSH (hypothyroidism)	• TSH levels above the upper limit of the normal range suggest an underactive thyroid (hypothyroidism) • Mildly elevated TSH levels (between 4.0 and 10.0 mIU/L) with normal levels of thyroxine (T4) may indicate subclinical hypothyroidism, especially if accompanied by symptoms (mild) and risk factors
	Decreased TSH (Hyperthyroidism)	• TSH levels below the lower limit of the normal range suggest an overactive thyroid (hyperthyroidism) • Low TSH levels are typically seen in conditions such as Graves' disease or toxic nodular goiter
Free Thyroxine (FT4)	Normal range	Typically between 0.8 to 1.8 ng/dL or 10 to 23 pmol/L
	Elevated FT4	High levels of FT4 may indicate hyperthyroidism
	Decreased FT4	Low levels of FT4 may indicate hypothyroidism

Type	Description	Range
Triiodothyronine (T3)	Normal range	• Typically between 80 to 200 ng/dL or 1.2 to 3.1 nmol/L • T3 levels are less commonly measured in routine thyroid panels but may be evaluated in specific clinical contexts

Interpretation

- Elevated TSH with normal or low FT4 levels suggests primary hypothyroidism, where the thyroid gland fails to produce enough thyroid hormones.
- Decreased TSH with elevated FT4 levels suggests primary hyperthyroidism, where the thyroid gland produces too much thyroid hormone.
- Subclinical hypothyroidism refers to mildly elevated TSH levels with normal FT4 levels. It is often temporary but may progress to overt hypothyroidism over time.
- Subclinical hyperthyroidism refers to mildly decreased TSH levels with normal FT4 levels. It may progress to overt hyperthyroidism or resolve spontaneously.
- Thyroid antibody tests (such as anti-thyroid peroxidase antibodies or anti-thyroglobulin antibodies) may be performed to evaluate for autoimmune thyroid diseases such as Hashimoto's thyroiditis or Graves' disease.

Chapter 27. Specialties Blood Test

A. ANA Test

> ➤ ANA (antinuclear antibody) testing is used to detect the presence of antibodies that target the body's own cell nuclei.
>
> ➤ Elevated ANA levels can indicate an autoimmune condition, but they can also be present in healthy patients or patients with non-autoimmune conditions.

Normal ANA levels

In healthy patients, ANA levels are typically low or undetectable. A negative ANA test result usually indicates that no significant autoimmune activity is present.

Elevated ANA levels

ANA levels are considered elevated when they are above a certain threshold, typically measured in titers (e.g., 1:80, 1:160, 1:320).

- Low-level elevations (e.g., 1:80): may be seen in healthy patients, especially older adults, and may not necessarily indicate autoimmune disease.
- Higher elevations (e.g., 1:160 or greater): are more likely to be associated with autoimmune conditions, but further evaluation is needed to determine the specific cause.

Interpretation in the context of symptoms and other tests

- ANA testing is not diagnostic of a specific autoimmune disease but rather indicates the presence of autoantibodies that may be associated with various conditions.
- The interpretation of ANA levels should be considered in the context of the patient's clinical presentation, medical history, and other laboratory findings.
- Additional tests, such as specific autoantibody tests (e.g., anti-dsDNA, anti-Smith antibodies) and clinical evaluation, are often needed to confirm a diagnosis of autoimmune disease.

Associated conditions

- Elevated ANA levels may be seen in a variety of autoimmune and non-autoimmune conditions, including systemic lupus erythematosus (SLE), Sjögren's syndrome, rheumatoid arthritis, scleroderma, autoimmune hepatitis, and others.

- ANA testing may also be positive in patients with infections, certain medications, cancer, or other non-autoimmune conditions.
- **Positive ANA and anti-histone antibodies** are classically associated with drug-induced lupus erythematosus (procainamide, hydralazine, etanercept, isoniazid...).

Follow-up and further evaluation
- If ANA levels are elevated, especially at moderate to high titers, further evaluation by a healthcare provider, typically a rheumatologist, is recommended.
- Additional tests and examinations may be performed to determine the underlying cause of the elevated ANA levels and to guide appropriate management and treatment.

The APhs should be aware that ANA testing alone is not sufficient for diagnosing autoimmune diseases. A thorough clinical evaluation, including medical history, physical examination, and additional laboratory tests, is necessary for accurate diagnosis and appropriate management.

The APh will interpret ANA test results in the context of a patient's overall health and recommend further evaluation or treatment if needed.

B. ESR/CRP Level

> ➤ *ESR (Erythrocyte Sedimentation Rate) and CRP (C-reactive Protein) are markers of inflammation commonly measured in blood tests.*

ESR (Erythrocyte Sedimentation Rate)

ESR measures the rate at which red blood cells settle in a tube of blood over time. It is a nonspecific marker of inflammation.

- Normal ESR: Values vary based on age and gender but are typically below 20 mm/hr for men and below 30 mm/hr for women.
- Elevated ESR: Elevated values indicate increased inflammation in the body but do not specify the cause.
    - Possible reasons for elevated ESR include infections, autoimmune diseases (such as rheumatoid arthritis or lupus), certain cancers, and other inflammatory conditions.

CRP (C-Reactive Protein)

CRP is a protein produced by the liver in response to inflammation. It is a more specific marker of acute inflammation compared to ESR.

- Normal CRP is typically below 10 mg/L, although the reference range may vary slightly between laboratories.
- Elevated CRP indicates acute inflammation in the body. CRP can rise dramatically in response to infections, tissue injury, autoimmune diseases, and other inflammatory conditions.

CRP levels can also be used to monitor response to treatment in certain conditions.

- A decrease in CRP levels over time may indicate improvement or resolution of inflammation.
- hs-CRP (high-sensitivity CRP) is usually elevated in patients with myocardial infarction; high levels of hs-CRP in otherwise healthy people are linked to an increased risk of future heart attack, stroke, sudden cardiac death and/or peripheral artery disease.

Interpretation

- Elevated ESR and CRP levels indicate the presence of inflammation in the body but do not provide specific information about the underlying cause.
- Further evaluation, including a thorough medical history, physical examination, and additional diagnostic tests, is often needed to determine the cause of inflammation.

- It's essential to interpret ESR and CRP levels in conjunction with other clinical findings and tests to guide diagnosis and treatment decisions accurately.

C. Lupus Panel

> ➤ *A lupus panel, also known as an autoimmune panel or connective tissue disease panel, is a blood test used to help diagnose systemic lupus erythematosus (SLE) and other autoimmune connective tissue diseases.*

Antinuclear Antibody (ANA, as explained above)

ANA is a marker of autoimmune activity.

- A positive ANA test suggests the presence of autoantibodies targeting the cell nuclei.
- ANA is not specific to lupus and can be positive in other autoimmune diseases and even in healthy patients.
- ANA testing is typically done using indirect immunofluorescence, and results are reported as titers (e.g., 1:80, 1:160, 1:320).

Anti-double-stranded DNA (anti-dsDNA) Antibodies

Anti-dsDNA antibodies specifically target double-stranded DNA and are more specific to lupus.

- Elevated levels of anti-dsDNA antibodies are strongly associated with active lupus and lupus nephritis (kidney involvement).

Anti-Sm Antibodies

Anti-Sm antibodies target a specific nuclear protein called the Smith (Sm) antigen. It has low sensitivity but high specificity for SLE.

- Anti-Sm antibodies are found in about 20-30% of patients with lupus, more commonly in African Americans and Asians than Causcasians.

Anti-Ro (SSA) and Anti-La (SSB) Antibodies

Anti-Ro and anti-La antibodies target the Ro and La proteins, respectively.

- These antibodies are associated with conditions such as Sjögren's syndrome and neonatal lupus (when passed from mother to fetus).

Anti-RNP Antibodies

Anti-RNP antibodies target the ribonucleoprotein (RNP) complex.

- Elevated levels of anti-RNP antibodies are associated with mixed connective tissue disease (MCTD) but can also be found in lupus and other autoimmune conditions.

Complement Levels (C3 and C4)

Complement proteins (C3 and C4) are part of the immune system and may be consumed in the presence of immune complex formation in lupus.
- Low levels of complement proteins may indicate lupus activity, especially if accompanied by other clinical manifestations.

Interpretation:
- A positive ANA test is often the first step in diagnosing lupus, but it is not sufficient on its own for a lupus diagnosis.
- The presence of anti-dsDNA antibodies, anti-Sm antibodies, or other lupus-specific antibodies supports the diagnosis of lupus, especially when accompanied by compatible clinical features.
- Complement levels may help assess disease activity, with low levels indicating complement consumption in active lupus.
- Interpretation of a lupus panel should consider the overall clinical picture, including symptoms, physical examination findings, and other laboratory tests.

Follow-Up
- A positive lupus panel may prompt further evaluation, including assessment for organ involvement (e.g., kidney, skin, joints) and monitoring disease activity over time.
- Additional tests or consultations with specialists (e.g., rheumatologists, nephrologists) may be needed to confirm the diagnosis and guide treatment decisions.

D. Rheumatoid Arthritis Panel

> *RF (Rheumatoid Factor) and anti-CCP (anti-Cyclic Citrullinated Peptide) antibodies are blood tests commonly used in the diagnosis and management of rheumatoid arthritis (RA) and other autoimmune rheumatic diseases.*

Rheumatoid Factor (RF)

RF is an autoantibody that targets the Fc portion of immunoglobulin G (IgG) antibodies.
- Elevated RF levels can be found in various autoimmune diseases, but they are most commonly associated with rheumatoid arthritis.
- RF positivity is found in a significant proportion of patients with RA, particularly those with seropositive RA.
- RF can also be positive in other conditions such as Sjögren's syndrome, systemic lupus erythematosus, and hepatitis C infection.

Anti-Cyclic Citrullinated Peptide (anti-CCP) Antibodies

Anti-CCP antibodies target citrullinated peptides, which are present in inflamed joints of patients with rheumatoid arthritis.

- Anti-CCP antibodies are highly specific to rheumatoid arthritis and are present in a significant proportion of patients with RA, especially those with early or aggressive disease.
- Anti-CCP positivity is associated with more severe disease and joint damage in RA.

Interpretation

- A positive RF or anti-CCP antibody test, especially in the presence of compatible clinical features, supports the diagnosis of rheumatoid arthritis.
- The presence of both RF and anti-CCP antibodies further increases the likelihood of rheumatoid arthritis, especially in patients with early or undifferentiated arthritis.
- However, it's important to note that RF and anti-CCP antibodies can also be present in other autoimmune and non-autoimmune conditions, and their presence alone is not diagnostic of rheumatoid arthritis.
- Interpretation of RF and anti-CCP antibody results should be done in the context of the overall clinical picture, including symptoms, physical examination findings, imaging studies, and other laboratory tests.

Follow-Up

A positive RF or anti-CCP antibody test may prompt further evaluation, including imaging studies (e.g., X-rays, ultrasound, MRI) and consultation with a rheumatologist.

- Additional tests or procedures may be needed to confirm the diagnosis, assess disease activity, and guide treatment decisions.

E. Cancer Markers

> ➤ *Cancer markers, also known as tumor markers, are substances produced by cancer cells or by the body in response to cancer.*
>
> ➤ *These markers can be detected in blood, urine, or tissue samples and are used for various purposes in cancer diagnosis, prognosis, monitoring, and treatment.*

Prostate-Specific Antigen (PSA)

- Used for screening and monitoring prostate cancer.

- Elevated PSA levels can indicate prostate cancer, but they can also be caused by non-cancerous conditions such as benign prostatic hyperplasia (BPH) or prostatitis.

CA 125

- Associated with ovarian cancer.
- Elevated CA 125 levels may indicate ovarian cancer, but they can also be elevated in other conditions such as endometriosis, pelvic inflammatory disease (PID), or uterine fibroids.

Carcinoembryonic Antigen (CEA)

- Associated with colorectal cancer and other gastrointestinal cancers.
- Elevated CEA levels can indicate colorectal cancer, but they can also be elevated in other cancers (e.g., pancreatic, lung) and non-cancerous conditions such as inflammatory bowel disease (IBD) or smoking.

Alpha-Fetoprotein (AFP)

- Associated with liver cancer (hepatocellular carcinoma) and certain types of germ cell tumors.
- Elevated AFP levels may indicate liver cancer, but they can also be elevated in other liver diseases (e.g., hepatitis, cirrhosis) and certain non-cancerous conditions.

CA 19-9

- Associated with pancreatic cancer and other gastrointestinal cancers.
- Elevated CA 19-9 levels may indicate pancreatic cancer, but they can also be elevated in other gastrointestinal cancers and non-cancerous conditions such as pancreatitis or biliary obstruction.

CA 15-3 and CA 27.29

- Associated with breast cancer.
- Elevated CA 15-3 and CA 27.29 levels may indicate breast cancer, particularly in advanced or metastatic disease, but they can also be elevated in other conditions.

CA 72-4

- Associated with gastrointestinal cancers, including stomach (gastric) cancer.
- Elevated CA 72-4 levels may indicate stomach cancer, but they can also be elevated in other gastrointestinal cancers and non-cancerous conditions.

HER2/neu (Human Epidermal Growth Factor Receptor 2)

- Associated with breast cancer and some other cancers.
- HER2/neu testing is used to determine the HER2 status of breast cancer tumors, which helps guide treatment decisions such as targeted therapy with drugs like trastuzumab (Herceptin).

AFP-L3%

- A subtype of alpha-fetoprotein associated with liver cancer (hepatocellular carcinoma).
- AFP-L3% testing can help differentiate between hepatocellular carcinoma and other liver conditions.

Ki-67

- A marker of cellular proliferation associated with various cancers.
- Ki-67 testing is used to assess tumor aggressiveness and predict response to treatment in certain cancers, including breast cancer and neuroendocrine tumors.

F. Vitamin D Level

> ➢ *Vitamin D is a fat-soluble vitamin crucial for calcium absorption in the gut, promoting bone health and playing a vital role in immune function, inflammation reduction, and muscle strength.*
>
> ➢ *Vitamin D is obtained through skin exposure to sunlight, certain foods (like fatty fish, fortified dairy products, and egg yolks), and dietary supplements.*
>
> ➢ *Insufficient vitamin D levels can lead to bone disorders such as rickets in children and osteoporosis in adults.*

25(OH)D Levels	Range	Description
Severe Deficiency	<10 ng/mL (25 nmol/L)	Symptoms of vitamin D deficiency may include muscle weakness, bone pain, fatigue, and an increased risk of fractures and osteoporosis
Deficiency	10-20 ng/mL (25-50 nmol/L)	
Insufficiency	21-29 ng/mL (50-74 nmol/L)	Some experts consider levels below 30 ng/mL (75 nmol/L) as insufficient for optimal health, as higher levels may provide additional benefits beyond bone health

25(OH)D Levels	Range	Description
Adequacy	30-100 ng/mL (75-250 nmol/L)	Levels above 30 ng/mL (75 nmol/L) are generally considered adequate for maintaining bone health and overall health, although optimal levels for other health outcomes are still debated
Optimal Range	40-60 ng/mL (100-150 nmol/L)	Patient requirements for vitamin D may vary based on factors such as age, ethnicity, geographic location, sun exposure, diet, and medical conditions
Toxicity	>150 ng/mL (375 nmol/L)	Vitamin D toxicity is rare but can occur with very high doses of supplementation, leading to elevated blood calcium levels (hypercalcemia) and symptoms such as nausea, vomiting, weakness, and kidney stones

Interpretation

- Interpretation of vitamin D levels should consider the patient's clinical context, including symptoms, risk factors for deficiency or insufficiency, and medical history.
- Testing may be indicated for patients with symptoms suggestive of vitamin D deficiency, those at higher risk (e.g., older adults, patients with limited sun exposure, certain medical conditions), or as part of routine health screening.
- The APh may recommend supplementation or lifestyle modifications (such as increased sun exposure and dietary changes) based on vitamin D levels and patient factors.
- Regular monitoring of vitamin D levels may be recommended for patients at risk of deficiency or insufficiency or those undergoing supplementation to ensure optimal levels and prevent potential adverse effects.

G. Vitamin B12 Level

> ➤ *Vitamin B12, also known as cobalamin, is essential for red blood cell formation, brain function, and DNA synthesis.*
>
> ➤ *It's naturally found in animal products, such as meat, fish, poultry, eggs, and dairy, with supplementation recommended for vegans or people with absorption issues.*
>
> ➤ *Deficiency in vitamin B12 can lead to anemia, neurological disorders, and cognitive impairments.*

Normal Range

- The normal range for serum vitamin B12 levels typically falls between 200 and 900 pg/mL or between 150 and 670 pmol/L. However, the reference range may vary slightly between laboratories.

Deficiency

- Vitamin B12 deficiency is typically defined as a serum B12 level below 200 pg/mL (148 pmol/L).
- Symptoms of vitamin B12 deficiency may include fatigue, weakness, numbness or tingling in the hands and feet, difficulty walking, memory problems, and mood changes.
- Severe deficiency can lead to pernicious anemia, neurological complications, and other health problems if left untreated.

Borderline Deficiency

- Serum B12 levels between 200 and 300 pg/mL (148-222 pmol/L) may be considered borderline deficient and may warrant further evaluation, especially if accompanied by symptoms or risk factors.

Elevated Levels

- Elevated vitamin B12 levels are less common but may occur in certain medical conditions such as liver disease, kidney failure, and myeloproliferative disorders.
- High levels of vitamin B12 are generally considered non-toxic, as excess B12 is usually excreted in the urine.

Interpretation

- Interpretation of vitamin B12 levels should consider the patient's clinical context, including symptoms, risk factors for deficiency, medical history, and other laboratory tests.
- Testing for vitamin B12 deficiency may be indicated in patients with symptoms suggestive of deficiency (such as fatigue, anemia,

neuropathy), those with conditions associated with malabsorption or impaired absorption of B12 (such as pernicious anemia, gastrointestinal disorders, or certain medications), or as part of routine health screening in older adults.

- Medications inhibit B12 absorption: metformin, colchicine, proton pump inhibitors, etc.
- Additional tests, such as methylmalonic acid (MMA) and homocysteine levels, may be used to further evaluate suspected vitamin B12 deficiency and differentiate between true deficiency and functional deficiency.
- Treatment for vitamin B12 deficiency typically involves oral or intramuscular supplementation with vitamin B12, depending on the underlying cause and severity of the deficiency.

H. Hemoglobin A1c and Blood Sugar Level

> *Hemoglobin A1c (HbA1c) measures the average blood sugar level over the past three months, reflecting the percentage of hemoglobin coated with sugar.*

Hemoglobin A1c (HbA1c) Interpretation
- Normal range: Less than 5.7%
- Prediabetes: 5.7% to 6.4%
- Diabetes: 6.5% or higher

Blood Sugar (Glucose) Interpretation

Fasting Plasma Glucose (FPG):
- Normal fasting glucose: Less than 100 mg/dL.
- Prediabetes (impaired fasting glucose): 100 to 125 mg/dL.
- Diabetes: 126 mg/dL or higher on two separate occasions.

Oral Glucose Tolerance Test (OGTT):
- Normal glucose tolerance: Less than 140 mg/dL two hours after the glucose load.
- Prediabetes: 140 to 199 mg/dL two hours after the glucose load.
- Diabetes: 200 mg/dL or higher two hours after the glucose load.

Random Plasma Glucose:
- Diabetes: 200 mg/dL or higher with classic symptoms of hyperglycemia.

- Note: Random glucose levels may not be reliable for diagnosing prediabetes.

Interpretation in Conjunction
- Elevated HbA1c levels, along with elevated fasting or postprandial glucose levels, indicate poor glycemic control and may suggest the need for treatment intensification or lifestyle modifications.
- HbA1c levels provide a long-term measure of glycemic control, while blood sugar measurements (FPG, OGTT, random glucose) offer a snapshot of glucose levels at specific times.
- Consistency between HbA1c and blood sugar measurements supports the reliability of the assessment of glycemic control.

Clinical Decision-Making
- The APh should use both HbA1c and blood sugar measurements to diagnose diabetes, assess glycemic control, and adjust treatment plans.
- Treatment goals are often based on both HbA1c targets and blood sugar measurements to reduce the risk of diabetes-related complications.
- Regular monitoring of HbA1c and blood sugar levels is essential for patients with diabetes to evaluate treatment efficacy and adjust management strategies as needed.

Patient Variability
- It's essential to consider patient variability and factors that may affect HbA1c and blood sugar measurements, such as age, ethnicity, comorbidities (kidney failure, liver disease, or severe anemia), medications, and adherence to treatment and monitoring regimens.

I. Uric Acid Level

> ➤ *Uric acid is a waste product formed from the breakdown of purines, substances found in various foods and drinks and naturally occurring in the body.*
>
> ➤ *Normally excreted in urine, elevated levels of uric acid can lead to gout, a form of arthritis characterized by painful joint inflammation, and can also be associated with kidney stones and renal failure.*
>
> ➤ *Management of high uric acid levels includes dietary changes, hydration, and medications to reduce production or increase excretion of uric acid.*

Normal Range
- The normal range for serum uric acid levels is typically:
  - For men: 3.4 to 7.0 mg/dL (200 to 420 µmol/L).
  - For women: 2.4 to 6.0 mg/dL (140 to 360 µmol/L).
- However, the reference range may vary slightly between laboratories.

Elevated Levels
- Elevated uric acid levels, known as hyperuricemia, may indicate increased production or decreased excretion of uric acid.
- Hyperuricemia can be caused by various factors, including dietary intake (high-purine foods), obesity, certain medications (e.g., thiazide diuretics), chronic kidney disease, metabolic syndrome, and genetic factors.
- Persistent hyperuricemia may increase the risk of developing gout, a type of arthritis caused by the deposition of urate crystals in the joints, as well as kidney stones and other health problems.

Low Levels
- Low uric acid levels are less common and may be seen in rare genetic disorders, certain medications (e.g., allopurinol), or conditions associated with increased excretion of uric acid (e.g., Fanconi syndrome).

Interpretation
- Interpretation of uric acid levels should consider the patient's clinical context, including symptoms, medical history, and other laboratory tests.
- Uric acid testing may be indicated in patients with symptoms suggestive of gout (e.g., sudden joint pain, swelling, redness), kidney stones, or other conditions associated with hyperuricemia.
- Elevated uric acid levels may prompt further evaluation to identify the underlying cause and assess the risk of developing gout or other complications.
- Treatment for hyperuricemia and gout may involve lifestyle modifications (e.g., dietary changes, weight loss), medications to reduce uric acid levels (e.g., allopurinol, febuxostat), and management of comorbidities such as hypertension and kidney disease.

Chapter 28. Other Tests

A. Protein and Urine Electrophoresis

> ➤ *Protein and urine electrophoresis are laboratory techniques used to separate and identify different proteins in the blood and urine, respectively, based on their size and charge.*
>
> ➤ *These tests are valuable in diagnosing and monitoring disorders such as multiple myeloma, chronic inflammatory conditions, and kidney diseases, by detecting abnormal levels and patterns of proteins.*
>
> ➤ *The results can help address specific protein abnormalities, guiding treatment decisions and monitoring disease progression or response to therapy.*

Total Protein in Urine
- Elevated total protein levels in urine, known as proteinuria, may indicate kidney damage or dysfunction, inflammation, infection, or systemic diseases affecting the kidneys.
- Proteinuria can be quantified as:
  - Trace or 1+ (mild proteinuria): 30 to 150 mg/dL.
  - 2+ (moderate proteinuria): 150 to 300 mg/dL.
  - 3+ (marked proteinuria): 300 to 1000 mg/dL.
  - 4+ (severe proteinuria): >1000 mg/dL.

Urinary Protein Electrophoresis
- Urinary protein electrophoresis separates and identifies different protein fractions in the urine, including albumin, globulins, and other proteins.
- The pattern of protein bands observed on the electrophoresis gel can provide insights into the underlying cause of proteinuria.
- Common patterns include increased albumin, increased alpha-2 globulins, and the presence of monoclonal bands.

Interpretation
- Interpretation of protein and urine electrophoresis results should consider the patient's clinical context, including symptoms, medical history, and other laboratory tests.
- Proteinuria may be transient or persistent and can be caused by various conditions such as glomerular diseases (e.g., nephrotic syndrome, glomerulonephritis), tubular disorders, urinary tract

infections, diabetes mellitus, hypertension, and systemic diseases (e.g., systemic lupus erythematosus, multiple myeloma).

- The pattern of protein bands observed on urine electrophoresis can help differentiate between different types of proteinuria and guide further diagnostic evaluation and management.

Follow-Up and Management

- Elevated total protein levels and abnormal protein patterns on urine electrophoresis may warrant further evaluation, including additional laboratory tests (e.g., serum protein electrophoresis, urine immunofixation), imaging studies, and kidney biopsy.
- Treatment for proteinuria depends on the underlying cause and may involve medications to control blood pressure, reduce inflammation, or treat underlying systemic diseases.
- Regular monitoring of proteinuria and urinary protein patterns may be necessary to assess treatment efficacy, disease progression, and kidney function.

B. Iron Panel

> ➢ *An iron panel evaluates iron levels in the body, including tests for serum iron, total iron-binding capacity (TIBC), transferrin saturation, and ferritin.*
>
> ➢ *It helps diagnose conditions like iron deficiency anemia or iron overload. Interpretation considers low or high levels of these markers, indicating potential iron-related disorders in the context of clinical findings.*

Test	Normal Range	Interpretation
Serum Iron	• 60-170 µg/dL (men) • 50-150 µg/dL (women)	Measures the amount of iron in the blood • Low levels may indicate iron deficiency • High levels may suggest iron overload

Test	Normal Range	Interpretation
Total Iron-Binding Capacity (TIBC)	240-450 µg/dL	Measures all proteins available to bind with iron, including transferrin • High levels often indicate iron deficiency, as the body produces more transferrin to try to capture more iron • Low levels may suggest iron overload or chronic illness
Transferrin Saturation	20-50%	Calculated by dividing serum iron by TIBC and multiplying by 100 • Low percentages (<20%) suggest iron deficiency • High percentages (>50%) indicate iron overload
Ferritin	• 20-500 ng/mL (men) • 20-200 ng/mL (women)	Reflects the amount of iron stored in the body • Low levels indicate iron deficiency • High levels may suggest iron overload or an acute phase reactant (indicative of inflammation)

Interpretation

- Iron Deficiency Anemia: Characterized by low serum iron, high TIBC, low transferrin saturation, and low ferritin.
- Anemia of Chronic Disease: May show normal or slightly low serum iron, low TIBC, normal or low transferrin saturation, and normal or high ferritin.
- Iron Overload (Hemochromatosis): Indicated by high serum iron, low TIBC, high transferrin saturation, and high ferritin.

C. Sex Hormones Panel

> ➤ A sex hormone panel evaluates hormones related to reproductive health, including estradiol, testosterone, follicle-stimulating hormone (FSH), luteinizing hormone (LH), and progesterone, to diagnose conditions like infertility, polycystic ovary syndrome (PCOS), and menopause.
>
> ➤ Normal ranges vary by sex, age, and, for women, the menstrual cycle phase.
>
> ➤ Interpretation should consider hormonal values and clinical symptoms to guide treatment strategies.

Sex Hormones	Gender	Range	Interpretation
Estradiol (E2)	Women	Levels vary significantly with the menstrual cycle: • Follicular phase: 30-120 pg/mL • Ovulatory peak: 130-370 pg/mL • Luteal phase: 70-250 pg/mL • Postmenopausal: <10-20 pg/mL	• High levels can indicate ovarian tumors or hyperstimulation • Low levels may suggest menopause or hypogonadism
	Men	10-50 pg/mL	High levels could be due to estrogen therapy, liver disease, or obesity
Testosterone	Women	15-70 ng/dL	High levels could suggest conditions like polycystic ovary syndrome (PCOS) or an adrenal or ovarian tumor
	Men	Normal range is typically 300-1,000 ng/dL (vary slightly depending on the lab)	Low levels may indicate hypogonadism

Sex Hormones	Gender	Range	Interpretation
Follicle-Stimu-lating Hormone (FSH)	Women	Varied by cycle phase: • Follicular phase : 5-20 IU/L • Mid-cycle peak: ~20-30 IU/L • Luteal phase: 1-10 IU/L • Postmenopausal: 30-120 IU/L	High levels can indicate menopause or diminished ovarian reserve
	Men	1-15 IU/L	• High levels may suggest testicular failure • Low levels could indicate problems with the pituitary gland or hypothalamus
Luteinizing Hormone (LH)	Women	Varied by cycle phase: • Follicular phase: 1-10 IU/L • Mid-cycle peak: ~10-60 IU/L • Luteal phase: 1-15 IU/L • Postmenopausal: 15-60 IU/L	• High LH levels are typical around ovulation and in conditions like PCOS • Low levels in both sexes could suggest hypopituitarism
	Men	1-15 IU/L	High levels may indicate primary testicular failure

Sex Hormones	Gender	Range	Interpretation
Progesterone	Women	Varied by cycle phase: • Follicular phase: <1 ng/mL • Mid-luteal phase: 5-20 ng/mL • Pregnant: >11 ng/mL, varies greatly with gestational age • Postmenopausal: <0.2 ng/mL	• Progesterone levels are used to confirm ovulation and assess placental and ovarian function during pregnancy • Low levels can indicate lack of ovulation or ectopic pregnancy
Sex Hormone-Bin-ding Globulin (SHBG)	Men	10-57 nmol/L	• High levels can decrease the availability of testosterone, leading to symptoms of hypogonadism despite normal total testosterone levels • Low levels can increase the availability of testosterone, potentially exacerbating conditions sensitive to androgens like PCOS
	Women	18-144 nmol/L	

C. Other Hormones Tests

Type	Hormone	Normal Range	Interpretation
Adrenal Hormone	Cortisol	10-20 µg/dL	• High levels may indicate Cushing's syndrome • Low levels suggest Addison's disease or secondary adrenal insufficiency
	ACTH	10-60 pg/mL	Levels are interpreted in conjunction with cortisol levels to assess adrenal and pituitary functions
	Insulin	<25 µIU/mL	High levels may indicate insulin resistance or early type 2 diabetes
Prolactin Hormone	Prolactin	• Women (non-pregnant): 2-29 ng/mL • Men: 2-18 ng/mL	Pregnant Women: Levels can rise significantly, up to 10-209 ng/mL or higher, especially in the third trimester

D. Hepatitis Panel

> ➤ *A hepatitis panel includes various markers to diagnose and monitor hepatitis A, B, and C infections, indicating acute or chronic infection, immunity, or the need for vaccination.*
>
> ➤ *Key markers include HBsAg and Anti-HBs for hepatitis B, Anti-HAV IgM/IgG for hepatitis A, and Anti-HCV and HCV RNA for hepatitis C.*
>
> ➤ *Interpretation depends on a combination of these markers to assess infection status, immunity, and infectivity.*

Hepatitis A
- Anti-HAV IgM: Indicates acute hepatitis A infection.
- Anti-HAV IgG: Indicates past infection and immunity to hepatitis A.

Hepatitis B
- HBsAg (Hepatitis B surface antigen): Indicates current hepatitis B infection. Persistent presence for more than six months suggests chronic infection.

- Anti-HBs (Hepatitis B surface antibody): Indicates recovery and immunity to hepatitis B. Can also indicate successful vaccination.
- Anti-HBc IgM (Hepatitis B core antibody, IgM): Indicates recent infection with hepatitis B, generally within the last 6 months.
- Anti-HBc IgG (Hepatitis B core antibody, IgG): Indicates past or ongoing infection with hepatitis B; can be present in those who have recovered or in those with chronic infection.
- HBeAg (Hepatitis B e antigen): Indicates active replication of the virus and high infectivity.
- Anti-HBe (Hepatitis B e antibody): Indicates a lower level of virus replication and reduced infectivity.

Hepatitis C

- Anti-HCV (Hepatitis C antibody): Indicates exposure to the hepatitis C virus. A positive result requires further testing with HCV RNA to determine if the infection is current.
- HCV RNA (Hepatitis C viral RNA): Indicates active hepatitis C infection. Quantitative tests measure the virus's load in the blood, important for treatment decisions and monitoring responses.

Hepatitis Interpretation

- Acute Hepatitis: Suggested by positive IgM antibodies for hepatitis A (Anti-HAV IgM) or hepatitis B (Anti-HBc IgM), or by the presence of HCV RNA for hepatitis C with or without Anti-HCV antibodies depending on the timing of testing post-exposure.
- Chronic Hepatitis: Indicated by the persistence of HBsAg for more than six months in hepatitis B, or by the presence of HCV RNA in hepatitis C without clearance over time.
- Immunity: Demonstrated by positive Anti-HAV IgG for hepatitis A, Anti-HBs for hepatitis B indicating recovery or successful vaccination, and the absence of Anti-HCV in the context of previous exposure without chronic infection development.
- Infectivity: Suggested by positive HBeAg for hepatitis B, indicating high viral replication and higher risk of transmission.

Tips to consider for the APh

- Confirmatory testing is essential for hepatitis C due to the possibility of false positives or past resolved infections.
- Chronic hepatitis B and C infections require careful monitoring for liver function and damage, as well as assessment for antiviral treatment eligibility.

- Vaccination history should be considered, especially for hepatitis B, as it can influence the interpretation of Anti-HBs.

E. Sexually Transmitted Disease Panel

> ➢ An STD panel is a comprehensive set of tests designed to screen for various sexually transmitted diseases, including HIV, syphilis, hepatitis B and C, herpes simplex virus, chlamydia, gonorrhea, and human papillomavirus (HPV).
>
> ➢ These tests help detect infections that may be asymptomatic and ensure timely treatment to prevent complications.
>
> ➢ Regular screening is recommended for sexually active individuals, especially those with new or multiple partners, to maintain sexual health and prevent disease transmission.

Disease	Test
HIV (Human Immunodeficiency Virus)	Antibody/antigen combination tests (4th generation tests), followed by confirmatory testing with Western blot or PCR for acute HIV infection
Syphilis	Non-treponemal tests (VDRL, RPR) for screening, followed by treponemal tests (FTA-ABS, TPPA) for confirmation
Hepatitis B	Surface antigen (HBsAg) to detect active infection, surface antibody (Anti-HBs) to assess immunity, and core antibody (Anti-HBc) to identify previous or ongoing infection
Hepatitis C	Anti-HCV antibody test followed by HCV RNA PCR tests for confirmation and to assess viral load
Herpes Simplex Virus	Type-specific serologic tests to detect antibodies to HSV-1 (oral herpes) and HSV-2 (genital herpes). PCR tests can be used for acute infection diagnosis
Chlamydia	Nucleic acid amplification tests (NAAT) from urine samples or swabs from genital areas, the throat, or the rectum
Gonorrhea	NAAT from urine samples or swabs from the urethra, cervix, throat, or rectum to detect Neisseria gonorrhoeae

Disease	Test
Human Papillomavirus (HPV)	High-risk HPV testing, often from cervical swab samples, especially for HPV types associated with the risk of cervical cancer

STD Interpretation

- Positive Results: Require confirmatory testing, clinical evaluation, and appropriate treatment. Partner notification and treatment may also be necessary to prevent reinfection and transmission.
- Negative Results: This may need to be repeated if testing occurs during the window period of an infection. Regular screening is recommended for sexually active individuals with new or multiple partners.

Prevention and Counseling

- Part of STD testing includes counseling on safe sex practices, the importance of regular screening, and, if necessary, vaccination (e.g., HPV and hepatitis B vaccines).

F. Prostate Panel

> *A prostate lab panel typically includes the Prostate-Specific Antigen (PSA) test to screen for prostate cancer, with elevated levels indicating the need for further evaluation.*
>
> *Additional tests like Free PSA, Prostate Health Index (PHI), and PCA3 may also be used to assess prostate cancer risk more accurately.*
>
> *These tests, combined with physical exams such as the Digital Rectal Exam (DRE), help diagnose and monitor prostate health conditions, guiding treatment decisions.*

Prostate-Specific Antigen (PSA)

- Purpose: Measures the level of PSA in the blood, a protein produced by both cancerous and noncancerous tissue in the prostate.
- Normal Range: Generally, a PSA level under 4 ng/mL is considered normal, but this can depend on age and race. Levels between 4-10 ng/mL are considered a gray area, and above 10 ng/mL is considered elevated.
- Interpretation:

- Elevated PSA levels can indicate prostate cancer, BPH, or prostatitis. However, PSA levels can also be influenced by age, prostate size, and other factors.
- The rate of PSA changes over time (PSA velocity) can also provide important diagnostic information.

Free PSA
- Purpose: Measures the percentage of PSA that is not bound to proteins in the blood. Used in conjunction with total PSA testing.
- Interpretation: A lower percentage of free PSA (<25%) might indicate a higher risk of prostate cancer in men with slightly elevated total PSA levels.

Digital Rectal Exam (DRE)
- Though not a lab test, the DRE is a physical exam that's often performed as part of prostate health screening.
- The APh feels the prostate through the rectal wall to check for bumps, soft or hard spots, and overall size and shape.

Additional Tests for Prostate Evaluation
- Prostate Health Index (PHI): Combines total PSA, free PSA, and [-2]proPSA levels for a more accurate assessment of prostate cancer risk.
- 4Kscore Test: Measures four prostate-specific biomarkers, providing a risk score for aggressive prostate cancer.
- PCA3 Test: A urine test after DRE that looks for the presence of the PCA3 gene in urine, which is overexpressed in prostate cancer cells.
- Transrectal Ultrasound (TRUS) and MRI: Imaging tests that provide visual images of the prostate, used for diagnosis and biopsy guidance.
- Prostate Biopsy: Recommended if other tests suggest the possibility of cancer. It involves collecting small samples of prostate tissue to look for cancer cells.

PSA Interpretation
- Elevated or borderline PSA levels often lead to further testing to determine the cause, which may include repeat PSA testing, imaging, or biopsy.
- The decision to proceed with more invasive testing like a biopsy should consider the patient's overall health, PSA level, DRE results, and personal preference.

Chapter 29. Basic EKG

> ➤ An EKG interpretation involves a systematic analysis of the waveform to evaluate the heart's electrical activity, structure, and function.
>
> ➤ This process can identify not only arrhythmias but also signs of cardiac ischemia, structural heart disease, electrolyte imbalances, and other conditions.

Rate and Rhythm

- Rate: Calculate the heart rate by counting the number of QRS complexes on the EKG strip (for a 6-second strip, multiply by 10; for other lengths, adjust accordingly).
- Rhythm: Determine if the rhythm is regular or irregular by measuring the intervals between consecutive QRS complexes.

P Wave Analysis

- Presence and Morphology: Confirm that there is a P wave before each QRS complex, indicating normal atrial depolarization. Assess for variations in shape, which may indicate atrial enlargement or ectopic atrial rhythms.
- P Wave Axis: The normal axis for P waves is between 0° and +75°, reflecting atrial depolarization from the SA node.

PR Interval

- Length: Measure the PR interval from the beginning of the P wave to the start of the QRS complex. The normal range is 0.12 to 0.20 seconds. Variations can indicate conduction delays or pre-excitation syndromes.

QRS Complex

- Duration: A normal QRS duration is up to 0.10 seconds. Longer durations may indicate bundle branch blocks or ventricular conduction abnormalities.
- Morphology: Evaluate for the presence of Q waves, which can indicate previous myocardial infarction and the overall morphology for signs of hypertrophy or conduction defects.

ST Segment and T Wave

- ST Segment: Analyze for elevation or depression, which may suggest myocardial ischemia, injury, or pericarditis.
- T Wave: Assess amplitude and direction. Inverted or peaked T waves can indicate ischemia, hyperkalemia, or other conditions.

QT Interval

- Measurement: From the start of the QRS complex to the end of the T wave, adjusting for heart rate. A prolonged QT interval increases the risk of torsades de pointes and other arrhythmias.

Axis Determination

- Frontal Plane Axis: Calculate the heart's electrical axis in the frontal plane by analyzing the QRS complex in limb leads. The normal axis is between -30° and +90°. Deviations can indicate underlying cardiac or pulmonary conditions.

Identification of Additional Features

- Look for other features such as premature beats, signs of chamber enlargement, and evidence of previous cardiac events.

References

- Briggs, C., Culp, N., Davis, B., & d'Onofrio, G. (2019). ICSH guidelines for the laboratory diagnosis of nonimmune hereditary red cell membrane disorders. International Journal of Laboratory Hematology, 41(S1), 24-37.
- Cervinski, M. A., Lee, H. K., & Martin, C. S. (2019). Clinical implications of pseudohyponatremia in a patient with hyperglycemia: A case report. BMC Endocrine Disorders, 19(1), 1-5.
- Wu, A. H. B., & Briggs, C. (2017). Assessment of glomerular filtration rate using urine measurements. In Laboratory Tests and Diagnostic Procedures (Vol. 1, pp. 1707-1710). John Wiley & Sons.
- Stone, N. J., Robinson, J. G., & et al. (2014). 2013 ACC/AHA guideline on the treatment of blood cholesterol to reduce atherosclerotic cardiovascular risk in adults: A report of the American College of Cardiology/American Heart Association Task Force on Practice Guidelines. Circulation, 129(25_suppl_2), S1-S45.
- Brent, G. A. (2012). Clinical practice. Graves' disease. New England Journal of Medicine, 358(24), 2594-2605.
- Hanly, J. G., & Pisetsky, D. S. (2010). Diagnosis and management of patients with antinuclear antibody-negative systemic lupus erythematosus. Best Practice & Research Clinical Rheumatology, 24(4), 531-542.
- McLean-Tooke, A., & Spickett, G. P. (2009). Association between antinuclear antibody and thrombosis: A case report and literature review. Rheumatology International, 29(12), 1493-1496.
- Hochberg, M. C. (1997). Updating the American College of Rheumatology revised criteria for the classification of systemic lupus erythematosus. Arthritis & Rheumatism, 40(9), 1725.
- Aletaha, D., Neogi, T., & et al. (2010). 2010 rheumatoid arthritis classification criteria: An American College of Rheumatology/European League Against Rheumatism collaborative initiative. Arthritis & Rheumatism, 62(9), 2569-2581.
- Duffy, M. J. (2013). Tumor markers in clinical practice: A review focusing on common solid cancers. Medical Principles and Practice, 22(1), 4-11.

- Holick, M. F. (2007). Vitamin D deficiency. New England Journal of Medicine, 357(3), 266-281.
- Langan, R. C., & Zawistoski, K. J. (2017). Update on vitamin B12 deficiency. American Family Physician, 89(12), 979-986.
- American Diabetes Association. (2020). 6. Glycemic targets: Standards of medical care in diabetes—2020. Diabetes Care, 43(Supplement 1), S66-S76.
- Richette, P., & Bardin, T. (2010). Gout. The Lancet, 375(9711), 318-328.
- Simerville, J. A., Maxted, W. C., & Pahira, J. J. (2005). Urinalysis: A comprehensive review. American Family Physician, 71(6), 1153-1162.

Part 4: When to Refer a Patient to the Specialist?

Chapter 30: General Principles of Referral in Primary Care

A. When to Refer A Patient to A Specialist?

Primary care providers (PCPs) play a central role in managing a broad range of medical conditions, but there are key moments when referring a patient to a specialist is necessary. Knowing **when to refer** can improve patient outcomes, expedite diagnosis, and ensure the patient receives the appropriate level of care.

1. **Criteria for Referral**:
    - **Uncertainty of Diagnosis**: When the PCP has exhausted initial diagnostic workup and is unsure of the underlying cause of symptoms, referral to a specialist is warranted. For instance, if a patient presents with atypical chest pain and preliminary tests (e.g., EKG, troponins) are inconclusive, a referral to a **cardiologist** for further diagnostic testing (e.g., stress test, coronary angiography) may be necessary.
        - According to a study in *JAMA*, timely referral when diagnosis is uncertain helps prevent diagnostic delays that could lead to worsened outcomes in conditions like **cancers**, **neurological disorders**, and **autoimmune diseases**.
    - **Failure of Standard Treatments**: When first-line treatments fail to control a patient's symptoms, referral to a specialist is often necessary to explore **advanced therapies**. For example, a patient with **type 2 diabetes** whose blood glucose remains uncontrolled despite the use of **oral hypoglycemics** may require referral to an **endocrinologist** for consideration of **insulin therapy** or other injectable agents.
        - Guidelines from the **American Diabetes Association (ADA)** emphasize referral in cases of persistent hyperglycemia after the failure of at least two classes of oral medications.
    - **Need for Specialized Tests or Treatments**: Many diagnostic tests, such as **colonoscopy**, **MRI-guided biopsies**, or **angiography**, require specialized skills and facilities. When such interventions are necessary, the PCP should refer the patient to a specialist capable of performing these procedures.
        - For example, a patient with **recurrent gastrointestinal bleeding** might need a **gastroenterology referral** for an endoscopic evaluation to rule out malignancies or inflammatory bowel disease.
2. **Communicating with Specialists**:
    - Effective communication with specialists is crucial to ensure seamless care. The **referral letter** or electronic note should contain key details to avoid duplicative testing and ensure efficient consultation.
    - **Essential information** to include in a referral letter:
        - **Patient's chief complaint** and relevant history.
        - **Initial diagnostic workup** performed in the primary care setting (e.g., labs, imaging).

- **Treatments attempted** and the patient's response.
- **Specific questions** or concerns the PCP wishes the specialist to address.
  - According to a study published in *BMJ Open*, clear and structured referral letters significantly improve communication between PCPs and specialists, leading to better patient outcomes and fewer unnecessary tests or delays in diagnosis.

B. Recognizing Red Flags Symptoms Across Systems

The ability to recognize **red flags**—signs or symptoms that suggest serious or life-threatening conditions—is one of the most important skills for PCPs. Early identification of critical symptoms ensures that patients with potentially serious diseases receive prompt evaluation and treatment, often by a specialist.

1. **The Importance of Early Identification of Critical Symptoms**:
   - **Red flags** symptoms are often subtle but can indicate serious pathology. The failure to recognize them can delay appropriate care, leading to **adverse outcomes**.
   - For example, recognizing the **red flag** of a sudden, severe headache in a patient with no prior history of migraines is essential, as this could suggest a **subarachnoid hemorrhage**. Immediate referral to **neurology** or **emergency services** for a **CT scan** or **lumbar puncture** is crucial for diagnosis and treatment.
   - Another common scenario is a patient presenting with **unexplained weight loss** and **night sweats**—symptoms that raise suspicion for **malignancy**, **tuberculosis**, or **HIV**. Recognizing these symptoms as red flags leads to timely referral for further testing.
2. **System-Based Overview of Red Flags in Common Conditions**:
   - **Cardiovascular System**: Chest pain radiating to the left arm or jaw, especially with associated **diaphoresis** and **shortness of breath**, suggests **acute coronary syndrome** and warrants urgent referral to a **cardiologist** or **emergency services**.
   - **Respiratory System**: A patient presenting with acute onset of **shortness of breath**, **pleuritic chest pain**, and **hemoptysis** could have a **pulmonary embolism**. Recognizing this red flag prompts immediate referral to **pulmonology** or the emergency department.
   - **Gastrointestinal System**: **Progressive dysphagia** with unintentional weight loss raises concerns for **esophageal cancer**, and early referral to a **gastroenterologist** for an endoscopy is indicated.
   - **Neurological System**: A **sudden, severe headache**, especially described as a "thunderclap," is a red flag for **subarachnoid hemorrhage**, and urgent imaging and referral to **neurology** are needed.

C. Balancing Management and Referral

While it is essential to refer patients when necessary, it is equally important for PCPs to manage conditions in the **primary care setting** whenever possible. This not only reduces healthcare costs but also allows for continuity of care and a more personal patient-doctor relationship.

1. **Managing Conditions in the Primary Care Setting Before Considering Referral**:
    - Many conditions can be managed initially in **primary care** with the application of **evidence-based guidelines**. For example, conditions such as **hypertension**, **type 2 diabetes**, and **hyperlipidemia** often respond well to lifestyle interventions and first-line medications, and referral should only be considered when these measures fail.
    - According to the **JNC 8 Hypertension Guidelines**, patients with **hypertension** should be referred to a **nephrologist** or **cardiologist** only after several failed attempts to control blood pressure with a combination of antihypertensive agents .
    - Another example is **low back pain**, which can often be managed with **conservative measures** (e.g., physical therapy, NSAIDs). Referral to an **orthopedic specialist** or **neurosurgeon** should be considered only if there are **red flags** (e.g., **cauda equina syndrome**, **progressive neurological deficits**).
2. **Co-Management Strategies with Specialists**:
    - **Co-management** between PCPs and specialists can be an effective approach for chronic conditions that require both primary and specialty care. For example, a PCP may continue managing a patient's **diabetes** in collaboration with an **endocrinologist**, especially in cases requiring **complex insulin regimens**.
    - Co-management works well in conditions like **chronic kidney disease (CKD)**. While early-stage CKD can be managed with lifestyle changes, blood pressure control, and **ACE inhibitors/ARBs** by the PCP, patients should be referred to a **nephrologist** for advanced CKD management or when **glomerular filtration rate (GFR)** declines below a certain threshold.
    - **Shared care models** have been shown to improve patient outcomes in conditions such as **heart failure**, where PCPs manage routine monitoring and medication adjustments while **cardiologists** focus on advanced interventions like **implantable defibrillators** or **transplant evaluations** .

References:

- Singh, H., et al. "Diagnostic Error in Medicine: Analysis of 583 Physician-Reported Errors." *JAMA*, 2018.
- American Diabetes Association. "Standards of Medical Care in Diabetes—2021." *Diabetes Care*, 2021.

- Tattersall, M. H., et al. "Referral Letters in Cancer Care: Why Are They Important?" *BMJ Open*, 2020.
- James, P. A., et al. "2014 Evidence-Based Guideline for the Management of High Blood Pressure in Adults: Report from the Panel Members Appointed to the Eighth Joint National Committee (JNC 8)." *JAMA*, 2014.
- Heneghan, C., et al. "Shared Care for Chronic Conditions: The Role of Generalists and Specialists." *British Medical Journal*, 2019.

Chapter 31: Cardiovascular Red Flags Symptoms

The cardiovascular system can present with a range of symptoms that require careful evaluation in primary care to determine when urgent referral is necessary. Early identification of **red flags** associated with life-threatening or progressive cardiovascular conditions can significantly impact patient outcomes.

Below is an elaboration on key cardiovascular red flags, their clinical implications, and when to refer to a **cardiologist**, **electrophysiologist**, or **emergency services**.

A. Chest Pain

1. **Red Flags for Chest Pain**:
    - **Sudden, severe chest pain**, especially when described as pressure-like or crushing, is a red flag for **acute coronary syndrome (ACS)**, which includes conditions such as **unstable angina, non-ST elevation myocardial infarction (NSTEMI)**, and **ST-elevation myocardial infarction (STEMI)**. These conditions require **emergency medical intervention** to prevent cardiac damage or death.
    - **Radiation of pain to the arm, jaw, or neck** is particularly concerning and is a classic sign of **cardiac ischemia**. Women may experience more **atypical presentations**, such as **nausea, back pain**, or **fatigue**, which should still be considered in the context of potential ACS.
    - **Shortness of breath** (dyspnea) and **diaphoresis** (sweating) accompanying chest pain further elevate suspicion for a cardiac origin. These symptoms suggest **poor cardiac perfusion** and **myocardial ischemia**.
    - Another important red flag is **sudden onset of tearing chest pain** that radiates to the back, which may indicate an **aortic dissection**, a life-threatening emergency requiring immediate surgical intervention.
    - Patients with risk factors for coronary artery disease (e.g., **hypertension, diabetes, hyperlipidemia, smoking history**) presenting with these symptoms should be referred immediately for further evaluation in an **emergency department** for potential thrombolysis, percutaneous coronary intervention (PCI), or surgery.
2. **When to Refer**:
    - Immediate referral to **emergency services** is warranted in any patient with suspected **acute coronary syndrome** or **aortic dissection**. These conditions require urgent diagnostic testing, such as **ECG, cardiac biomarkers** (troponin), and potentially **CT angiography** for aortic dissection.
    - Referral to a **cardiologist** is necessary for patients with **chronic chest pain** that is suggestive of **stable angina**, particularly if it is triggered by exertion and relieved by rest. These patients may require stress testing, echocardiography, or **coronary angiography** to further evaluate coronary artery disease.
    - According to the **American College of Cardiology (ACC)** guidelines, patients with **stable chest pain** but at high risk for cardiac disease should be referred for

outpatient cardiology consultation for further management and possible revascularization .

B. Hypertension

1. **Red Flags for Hypertension**:
   - **Resistant hypertension** is defined as blood pressure that remains above the goal despite the use of **three or more antihypertensive medications**, including a diuretic. This may indicate an underlying condition, such as **secondary hypertension** (e.g., **renal artery stenosis, pheochromocytoma, primary aldosteronism**), and requires referral for further evaluation.
   - **Hypertensive emergencies** are characterized by severe elevations in blood pressure (typically **>180/120 mm Hg**) accompanied by signs of **end-organ damage**, such as **acute kidney injury, retinopathy, heart failure**, or **stroke**. Patients may present with **headaches, vision changes, chest pain**, or **neurological deficits**.
   - **Secondary hypertension indicators** include symptoms suggestive of underlying causes such as **unexplained hypokalemia** (suggesting hyperaldosteronism), **paroxysmal sweating, palpitations**, and **headaches** (suggesting pheochromocytoma), or **bruits** on physical examination (suggesting renovascular disease).
2. **When to Refer**:
   - Referral to a **nephrologist** is indicated for patients with suspected **renal artery stenosis, chronic kidney disease**, or **other secondary causes** of hypertension. Nephrologists can perform advanced diagnostic testing, such as **renal ultrasound with Doppler** or **renal angiography**, to assess the renal vasculature.
   - **Cardiologist referral** is recommended when a patient's hypertension is complicated by **heart failure, left ventricular hypertrophy**, or if there is concern for **coronary artery disease**. Cardiologists may consider additional tests like **echocardiography** or **ambulatory blood pressure monitoring** to further investigate the extent of organ damage or refractory hypertension.
   - Hypertensive emergencies require **emergency department referral** for **intravenous antihypertensives** and continuous monitoring to prevent further end-organ damage, following guidelines from the **American Heart Association (AHA)**.

C. Palpitations and Arrhythmias

1. **Red Flags for Palpitations and Arrhythmias**:

- **Syncope** (fainting) or **near-syncope** associated with palpitations is a significant red flag. It may indicate **serious arrhythmias**, such as **ventricular tachycardia** or **bradyarrhythmias** (e.g., heart block), which increase the risk of sudden cardiac death.
- **Irregular rhythm** associated with **dizziness**, **fatigue**, or **shortness of breath** may be a sign of **atrial fibrillation** or other supraventricular arrhythmias. These arrhythmias increase the risk of **thromboembolic events** like **stroke** and require early identification and management.
- **Atrial fibrillation** is often asymptomatic but can present with **palpitations** or **fatigue**. It is critical to assess patients for **hemodynamic instability** and risk factors for stroke using tools such as the **CHA2DS2-VASc score**, which helps guide the need for **anticoagulation** therapy.

2. **When to Refer**:
   - Referral to a **cardiologist** or **electrophysiologist** is indicated for patients with **symptomatic palpitations**, particularly when they occur in the context of **syncope** or with signs of **hemodynamic instability**. Cardiac monitoring via **Holter monitors**, **event recorders**, or **implantable loop recorders** may be necessary to capture intermittent arrhythmias.
   - Patients with **atrial fibrillation** should be referred for further evaluation to determine the need for **rate control** or **rhythm control** strategies. In some cases, patients may be candidates for **catheter ablation** or **electrical cardioversion**.
   - Urgent referral or emergency evaluation is warranted in patients with **syncope** and palpitations, as these may suggest life-threatening arrhythmias like **ventricular tachycardia**. **Implantable cardioverter-defibrillators (ICDs)** may be considered in patients at high risk of sudden cardiac death.
   - According to the **American College of Cardiology (ACC)/American Heart Association (AHA) guidelines**, patients with **atrial fibrillation** and high thromboembolic risk should be referred for **anticoagulation** assessment, and if necessary, for **cardioversion** or **ablation procedures**.

Recognizing red flags in cardiovascular conditions is critical for primary care physicians. **Chest pain**, **hypertension**, and **arrhythmias** each carry the risk of severe complications, including **myocardial infarction**, **stroke**, and **sudden cardiac death**.

Timely referrals to **cardiologists**, **electrophysiologists**, or **emergency services** based on these red flags ensure patients receive the specialized care they need and improve overall outcomes.

References

1. Amsterdam, E. A., et al. "2014 AHA/ACC Guideline for the Management of Patients With Non–ST-Elevation Acute Coronary Syndromes." *Journal of the American College of Cardiology*, 2014.

2. Whelton, P. K., et al. "2017 ACC/AHA Hypertension Guidelines: A Systematic Review for the U.S. Preventive Services Task Force." *Annals of Internal Medicine*, 2017.
3. January, C. T., et al. "2019 AHA/ACC/HRS Guideline for the Management of Patients With Atrial Fibrillation." *Circulation*, 2019.
4. Mancia, G., et al. "ESH/ESC Guidelines for the Management of Arterial Hypertension." *European Heart Journal*, 2018.
5. Zipes, D. P., et al. "ACC/AHA/ESC 2006 Guidelines for the Management of Patients With Ventricular Arrhythmias and the Prevention of Sudden Cardiac Death." *Journal of the American College of Cardiology*, 2006.

Chapter 32: Respiratory Red Flags Symptoms

Respiratory complaints such as **shortness of breath**, **cough**, and **wheezing** are common in primary care, but the presence of certain **red flags** can indicate serious underlying pathology requiring urgent intervention or specialist referral.

Recognizing these red flags is critical to avoid delayed diagnosis and treatment of life-threatening conditions. Below is a detailed overview of respiratory red flags, with recommendations on when to refer to **pulmonology** or **emergency services**.

A. Shortness of Breath (Dyspnea)

1. **Red Flags for Shortness of Breath**:
    - **Acute onset of dyspnea** is a critical red flag that may indicate serious, life-threatening conditions such as:
        - **Pulmonary embolism (PE)**: Sudden onset of **dyspnea**, often associated with **pleuritic chest pain**, **tachycardia**, or **hemoptysis**. Risk factors include **recent surgery**, **immobility**, **oral contraceptive use**, or a history of **deep vein thrombosis (DVT)**. PE is a medical emergency due to the risk of **right heart failure** and death from occlusion of the pulmonary arteries.
        - **Pneumothorax**: Sudden onset of **unilateral pleuritic chest pain** and **dyspnea**, often accompanied by **decreased breath sounds** and **hyperresonance** on the affected side. Spontaneous pneumothorax can occur in healthy individuals, particularly in tall, thin males, but is more common in those with underlying **chronic obstructive pulmonary disease (COPD)** or **cystic fibrosis**. If untreated, it can progress to a **tension pneumothorax**, leading to cardiovascular collapse.
        - **Asthma exacerbation**: Sudden worsening of dyspnea, with associated **wheezing**, **cough**, and **chest tightness**, can signify an acute asthma attack. **Status asthmaticus**, or a severe asthma attack unresponsive to standard treatments, can lead to respiratory failure.
2. **When to Refer**:
    - **Immediate referral to emergency services** is required for suspected **pulmonary embolism, pneumothorax**, or **status asthmaticus**, as these conditions can rapidly progress to respiratory or cardiovascular collapse. Emergency imaging (e.g., **CT pulmonary angiography** for PE, **chest X-ray** for pneumothorax) and interventions (e.g., **anticoagulation, needle decompression, bronchodilators**) are crucial.
    - **Pulmonology referral** is indicated for chronic dyspnea of unclear etiology, particularly when associated with conditions such as **interstitial lung disease**, **COPD**, or **pulmonary hypertension**. Pulmonologists can perform specialized testing such as **pulmonary function tests (PFTs)** and **high-resolution CT** to determine the underlying cause of chronic dyspnea.

Clinical Relevance:
Pulmonary embolism is a major cause of sudden death if left untreated, with mortality rates of up to 30% without intervention. Early identification and treatment with **anticoagulation** or **thrombolytics** are essential for improving outcomes. Similarly, **tension pneumothorax** and **status asthmaticus** require rapid intervention to prevent fatal complications .

B. Cough

1. **Red Flags for Cough**:
   - A **persistent cough lasting more than 8 weeks** is classified as chronic and requires further investigation, particularly when associated with red flags such as:
     - **Hemoptysis**: Coughing up blood is concerning for **lung cancer**, **tuberculosis (TB)**, or severe **bronchiectasis**. Even small amounts of blood in the sputum should prompt urgent evaluation, as lung cancer often presents initially with hemoptysis.
     - **Unexplained weight loss** and **night sweats**: These symptoms, when associated with a chronic cough, raise concerns for **lung cancer**, **tuberculosis**, or other systemic illnesses such as **lymphoma**. Tuberculosis should be suspected in high-risk individuals, such as those with **HIV**, **immunosuppressive therapy**, or recent travel to endemic regions.
     - **Purulent sputum** and **dyspnea**: These can indicate chronic infections like **bronchiectasis** or advanced **COPD**, where recurrent infections can cause progressive lung damage.
2. **When to Refer**:
   - **Referral to pulmonology** is indicated for patients with a **persistent cough** and any associated red flags such as hemoptysis, weight loss, or night sweats. Pulmonologists can perform further investigations, including **bronchoscopy**, **CT imaging**, and **sputum cultures**, to rule out malignancies, tuberculosis, or other infections.
   - **Immediate referral** is warranted for patients presenting with large-volume hemoptysis, as this may require **bronchial artery embolization** or surgical intervention to control bleeding.

Clinical Relevance:
Lung cancer is the leading cause of cancer-related deaths worldwide, and persistent cough is often an early symptom. Early recognition of red flags associated with lung cancer, such as hemoptysis and weight loss, can lead to timely diagnosis and intervention. **Tuberculosis** remains a global health concern, with nearly 10 million cases reported annually, emphasizing the need for prompt referral and isolation precautions in high-risk patients .

C. Wheezing and Stridor

1. **Red Flags for Wheezing and Stridor**:
    - **Acute wheezing unresponsive to bronchodilators** is a significant red flag for conditions such as **status asthmaticus** or severe **bronchospasm** in COPD. Patients may present with worsening dyspnea, **chest tightness**, and minimal improvement with standard therapies, indicating a need for escalation of care.
    - **Stridor**, a high-pitched sound heard during inspiration, indicates **upper airway obstruction**. It may result from:
        - **Anaphylaxis**, presenting with **wheezing, stridor**, and **facial swelling**, is a life-threatening allergic reaction that requires immediate administration of **epinephrine**.
        - **Foreign body aspiration**, common in children, presents with **sudden onset of stridor** or wheezing and requires emergency evaluation.
        - **Epiglottitis**, an infection of the epiglottis, presents with **fever, drooling**, and **stridor** in both children and adults. It requires urgent airway management and intravenous antibiotics.
2. **When to Refer**:
    - **Urgent referral to emergency services** is required for patients with **audible stridor** or **wheezing** that is unresponsive to bronchodilators. These conditions, particularly if associated with **cyanosis, altered mental status**, or impending respiratory failure, may require **intubation, tracheostomy**, or other advanced airway management.
    - Referral to **pulmonology** is indicated for chronic or recurrent **wheezing** to evaluate for underlying conditions such as **asthma, COPD**, or **vocal cord dysfunction**. Pulmonologists may use tools such as **spirometry, bronchoscopy**, or **laryngoscopy** to assess airway dynamics and obstruction.

Clinical Relevance:
Stridor is a hallmark of **upper airway obstruction** and requires immediate attention to prevent airway collapse. Conditions such as **anaphylaxis** and **foreign body aspiration** are medical emergencies, with mortality risks if left untreated. Similarly, **status asthmaticus** is a life-threatening asthma exacerbation that necessitates aggressive management, including **intravenous steroids, magnesium sulfate**, and, in some cases, mechanical ventilation.

References

- Wells, P. S., et al. "Diagnosis of pulmonary embolism: a clinical and imaging challenge." *Journal of the American College of Cardiology*, 2021.
- Marcus, M. B., et al. "Lung cancer screening: an update and implications for primary care." *Annals of Internal Medicine*, 2019.
- Castro-Rodriguez, J. A., et al. "Predictors of wheezing and asthma in childhood: A systematic review." *Allergy*, 2018.
- Kessler, C., et al. "Wheezing and stridor: Evaluation and management in the emergency department." *Emergency Medicine Clinics of North America*, 2020.

- Global Initiative for Asthma (GINA). "Global Strategy for Asthma Management and Prevention." *GINA Report*, 2021.

Chapter 33: Gastrointestinal Red Flags

Gastrointestinal (GI) symptoms such as **abdominal pain**, **dysphagia**, and **rectal bleeding** are common in clinical practice. However, the presence of certain **red flags** can indicate serious, potentially life-threatening conditions that require urgent referral to **gastroenterology** or **general surgery**.

Recognizing these red flags and acting promptly is critical for preventing complications and improving patient outcomes. Below is a summary on the key GI red flags and when to refer to specialists.

A. Abdominal Pain

1. **Red Flags for Abdominal Pain**:
   - **Severe, sudden abdominal pain** is a significant red flag, especially in the elderly. Acute, intense pain associated with **guarding, rebound tenderness**, or signs of **peritoneal irritation** may indicate a surgical emergency such as:
     - **Appendicitis**: Presents with **acute, localized pain** in the **right lower quadrant** (RLQ), often starting near the umbilicus and migrating to the RLQ. Guarding, rebound tenderness, and positive **McBurney's sign** are classic physical exam findings. **Fever, anorexia**, and **elevated white blood cell count** may accompany these symptoms.
     - **Bowel perforation**: Characterized by **sudden, severe pain** and signs of **peritonitis** (rigid abdomen, rebound tenderness). Causes include **peptic ulcer perforation, diverticulitis**, or **trauma**. **Free air** under the diaphragm on abdominal X-ray or CT scan is a hallmark of perforation.
     - **Mesenteric ischemia**: This life-threatening condition typically presents with **sudden onset severe abdominal pain** that is disproportionate to physical findings. It is most common in elderly patients with **atrial fibrillation** or other risk factors for embolism or thrombosis. Untreated, mesenteric ischemia can lead to bowel necrosis and sepsis.
2. **When to Refer**:
   - **Immediate referral to general surgery** is required for patients presenting with **acute abdominal pain** associated with **peritoneal signs** (guarding, rebound tenderness) or signs of **shock** (hypotension, tachycardia), as these symptoms suggest a need for **emergency surgical intervention**. Conditions like **appendicitis, bowel perforation**, or **mesenteric ischemia** are surgical emergencies.
   - Referral to **gastroenterology** is warranted for patients with less acute, but persistent or recurrent abdominal pain, particularly if it is associated with **systemic symptoms** like weight loss or GI bleeding. Gastroenterologists may perform diagnostic tests such as **endoscopy** or **colonoscopy** to further investigate non-surgical causes of abdominal pain.

3. **Clinical Significance**:
   Delayed recognition of **mesenteric ischemia** is associated with a high mortality rate, with studies indicating that outcomes improve significantly with early surgical intervention. Similarly, rapid diagnosis and surgical treatment of **appendicitis** and **bowel perforation** are crucial to prevent complications like peritonitis and sepsis.

B. Dysphagia (Difficulty Swallowing)

1. **Red Flags for Dysphagia**:
   - **Progressive dysphagia** (difficulty swallowing that worsens over time) is a major red flag, particularly when associated with **weight loss, pain,** or **regurgitation**. This symptom pattern is highly suggestive of an obstructive lesion in the esophagus, such as:
     - **Esophageal cancer**: Presents with **progressive dysphagia** to solids initially, then to liquids, accompanied by **unintentional weight loss**, **chest pain**, or **odynophagia** (painful swallowing). Esophageal cancer is often diagnosed at an advanced stage, so early recognition is critical.
     - **Achalasia**: A rare motility disorder that causes **progressive dysphagia** to both solids and liquids due to failure of the lower esophageal sphincter to relax. Patients may experience **regurgitation** of undigested food, **chest pain**, and **weight loss**.
     - **Esophageal strictures**: These can be caused by chronic **gastroesophageal reflux disease (GERD)**, radiation therapy, or **caustic ingestion** and present with progressive dysphagia. Unlike cancer, strictures usually cause no pain but can still lead to significant malnutrition if untreated.
2. **When to Refer**:
   - Referral to **gastroenterology** is required for any patient presenting with **progressive dysphagia**, especially if associated with **weight loss** or **chest pain**. Urgent evaluation with **upper endoscopy (EGD)** is necessary to rule out **esophageal cancer** or other structural abnormalities. If malignancy is suspected, **biopsies** should be taken during endoscopy to confirm the diagnosis.
   - For cases of suspected **achalasia** or motility disorders, additional testing such as **esophageal manometry** may be required, and gastroenterologists can guide treatment options, including **pneumatic dilation**, **Heller myotomy**, or **botulinum toxin injections**.
3. **Clinical Significance**:
   Early diagnosis of **esophageal cancer** significantly improves survival rates, with 5-year survival rates ranging from 15% to 20% depending on the stage at diagnosis. Delayed recognition can lead to advanced disease, making curative treatment difficult. Dysphagia associated with weight loss or pain should always prompt urgent referral for endoscopic evaluation.

C. Rectal Bleeding

1. **Red Flags for Rectal Bleeding**:
   - **Bright red blood per rectum (hematochezia)** or **melena** (black, tarry stools) are concerning signs of **gastrointestinal bleeding**. When associated with **anemia**, **fatigue**, or **weight loss**, rectal bleeding raises concerns for:
     - **Colorectal cancer**: A common cause of **rectal bleeding** in older adults, often associated with **iron-deficiency anemia**, **unexplained weight loss**, and **changes in bowel habits** (e.g., alternating constipation and diarrhea). Any patient over 50 with new-onset rectal bleeding or changes in stool caliber should be evaluated for colorectal cancer.
     - **Diverticular disease**: Bleeding from **diverticula** can be painless and present as sudden, large-volume rectal bleeding in elderly patients.
     - **Gastrointestinal (GI) bleed**: Upper GI bleeding (e.g., peptic ulcer disease, esophageal varices) can present as **melena** due to the presence of partially digested blood in the stool. **Lower GI bleeding** typically causes **hematochezia** and may be due to **hemorrhoids**, **diverticulitis**, or **angiodysplasia**.
     - **Inflammatory bowel disease (IBD)**: Patients with **Crohn's disease** or **ulcerative colitis** may present with **rectal bleeding**, often associated with **abdominal pain**, **diarrhea**, and **weight loss**.
2. **When to Refer**:
   - Referral to **gastroenterology** for **colonoscopy** is essential for patients presenting with **rectal bleeding**, especially if associated with **anemia**, **weight loss**, or **abdominal pain**. Colonoscopy allows for direct visualization of the colon and rectum and enables **biopsy** of suspicious lesions.
   - **Urgent referral** to **gastroenterology** or **emergency services** is required for patients with significant **acute GI bleeding** resulting in hemodynamic instability (hypotension, tachycardia), as this may necessitate **endoscopic intervention** or **transfusion**.
3. **Clinical Significance**:
   Colorectal cancer is the third most common cancer worldwide, and early detection through colonoscopy can prevent progression and improve survival. In cases of **acute GI bleeding**, rapid assessment and intervention are crucial to prevent shock and further complications. **Diverticular bleeding**, while common, can also result in significant blood loss and often requires endoscopic management or surgery.

Chapter 34: Neurological Red Flags Symptoms

Neurological symptoms such as **headache**, **dizziness**, and **seizures** are common complaints in clinical practice. However, when associated with specific **red flags**, they may indicate life-threatening or progressive neurological conditions.

Early identification and prompt referral to **neurology**, **epileptology**, or **emergency services** are critical for improving patient outcomes. Below is a summary on key neurological red flags, their clinical implications, and referral recommendations.

A. Headache

1. **Red Flags for Headache**:
   - **Sudden onset headache** (often referred to as a **thunderclap headache**) is a significant red flag that can indicate a **subarachnoid hemorrhage (SAH)** or **stroke**. Patients often describe the pain as the "worst headache of my life," with rapid onset and peak intensity within seconds to minutes. A **ruptured cerebral aneurysm** is a common cause of SAH, which can lead to permanent brain damage or death if not recognized and treated quickly.
   - Headaches associated with **neurological deficits**, such as **weakness**, **visual disturbances**, or **aphasia**, raise suspicion for an acute **ischemic stroke** or **intracranial hemorrhage**.
   - **Visual changes** (e.g., blurred vision, loss of vision), particularly if accompanied by a headache, may suggest **giant cell arteritis** or **increased intracranial pressure** due to a brain tumor or **venous sinus thrombosis**.
   - **Vomiting**, especially without nausea, in the context of a severe headache could indicate **elevated intracranial pressure** caused by a **space-occupying lesion** or **intracranial hemorrhage**.
2. **When to Refer**:
   - **Immediate referral to emergency services** is warranted for patients presenting with a **sudden-onset thunderclap headache**, as this may indicate **subarachnoid hemorrhage** or **stroke**. **CT imaging** of the head is typically the first step in diagnosing these conditions, and **lumbar puncture** may be necessary if imaging is inconclusive but clinical suspicion for SAH remains high.
   - Referral to **neurology** is appropriate for patients with **chronic or recurrent headaches** associated with **neurological symptoms**, **visual disturbances**, or **systemic symptoms** like **weight loss** (e.g., giant cell arteritis). **MRI** of the brain or **angiography** may be required for further evaluation.
3. **Clinical Significance**:
   Subarachnoid hemorrhage accounts for 5% of all strokes and carries a mortality rate of approximately 50%, emphasizing the need for rapid diagnosis and intervention. Early referral and treatment of **stroke** or **space-occupying lesions** can prevent permanent neurological damage and improve long-term outcomes.

B. Dizziness and Vertigo

1. **Red Flags for Dizziness and Vertigo**:
   - **Acute onset dizziness or vertigo** with associated **neurological symptoms** such as **diplopia** (double vision), **ataxia** (impaired coordination), or **weakness** is concerning for **posterior circulation stroke** or **brainstem pathology**. These areas of the brain control balance and coordination, and strokes in these regions may be initially misdiagnosed as benign vertigo or inner ear disorders.
     - **Stroke** in the **posterior circulation** (e.g., vertebrobasilar system) can present with **vertigo, gait instability**, and **dysarthria** (slurred speech). The **HINTS exam** (Head Impulse, Nystagmus, Test of Skew) can help differentiate between central causes (e.g., stroke) and peripheral causes (e.g., benign positional vertigo).
   - **Positional changes** that trigger dizziness with **neurological symptoms** such as **weakness** or **visual disturbances** may indicate an underlying **brainstem lesion** or **cerebellar infarct**.
   - **Severe vertigo** with hearing loss and tinnitus may suggest **Meniere's disease** but should be differentiated from a more serious central cause of vertigo, such as a stroke or mass lesion.
2. **When to Refer**:
   - Patients presenting with **acute onset dizziness or vertigo** accompanied by **neurological symptoms** (e.g., **diplopia, ataxia**, or **weakness**) should be referred immediately to **emergency services** for evaluation of possible **stroke** or **brainstem pathology**. MRI of the brain is often necessary to rule out stroke or other central causes.
   - Referral to **neurology** is appropriate for chronic or recurrent vertigo with concerning features, or when a **central cause** is suspected. Neurologists may perform **vestibular function testing**, MRI, or **angiography** to evaluate the underlying etiology.
3. **Clinical Significance**:
   Posterior circulation strokes can be easily missed, as their symptoms (dizziness, vertigo, and ataxia) often mimic benign conditions. Failure to diagnose can result in significant morbidity or death. Studies show that the **HINTS exam** can help distinguish between central and peripheral causes of vertigo, significantly improving diagnostic accuracy in the acute setting.

C. Seizures

1. **Red Flags for Seizures**:
   - **New onset of seizures in adults**, especially in patients with no prior history of seizures, is concerning for an underlying structural lesion such as a **brain tumor**,

- **stroke**, or **meningitis**. Any new seizure in an adult should prompt urgent evaluation to rule out these causes.
  - **Prolonged postictal confusion** following a seizure (lasting hours rather than minutes) may suggest **focal neurological damage** or **metabolic abnormalities**, and requires further investigation.
  - **Associated focal neurological deficits** (e.g., weakness, sensory changes) following a seizure raise concerns for **brain tumors**, **vascular malformations**, or **stroke**. These deficits may be subtle but signify an underlying structural lesion.
  - **Status epilepticus**, defined as a seizure lasting more than five minutes or repeated seizures without recovery in between, is a neurological emergency that requires immediate intervention to prevent permanent brain damage.
2. **When to Refer**:
   - **Immediate referral to emergency services** is indicated for any patient with **status epilepticus**, as this condition requires **intravenous anticonvulsants** and close monitoring to prevent brain damage or death.
   - Patients with **new-onset seizures** or seizures associated with **focal deficits** should be referred to **neurology** or **epileptology** for further evaluation. **MRI of the brain** and **electroencephalography (EEG)** are critical for diagnosing the cause of seizures and guiding treatment.
   - Referral to **epileptology** is also recommended for patients with **recurrent seizures** despite treatment, as they may benefit from specialized care, including medication adjustments, **vagal nerve stimulation**, or **surgical interventions** for refractory epilepsy.
3. **Clinical Significance**:

New-onset seizures in adults often signal an underlying **structural brain lesion**, such as a **tumor** or **stroke**. Delayed diagnosis of these conditions can result in worsening neurological outcomes. Additionally, **status epilepticus** carries a high risk of mortality and requires immediate treatment. **Brain tumors** are often discovered in the workup of new seizures, making early referral and imaging crucial for diagnosis and management.

References

- Linn, F. H., et al. "Subarachnoid hemorrhage: Diagnostic challenges in primary care." *Journal of Neurology*, 2020.
- Newman-Toker, D. E., et al. "Dizziness and vertigo in the emergency department." *New England Journal of Medicine*, 2021.
- Fisher, R. S., et al. "Epileptic seizures and epilepsy: Definitions and classification." *Epilepsia*, 2020.
- Saber Tehrani, A. S., et al. "Posterior circulation stroke: A diagnostic challenge for emergency physicians." *The Journal of Emergency Medicine*, 2020.
- Rosenow, F., et al. "New-onset seizures and epilepsy in the elderly: Diagnostic considerations." *Journal of Neurology, Neurosurgery & Psychiatry*, 2019.

Chapter 35: Musculoskeletal Red Flags

Musculoskeletal complaints such as **back pain, joint pain**, and **trauma-related injuries** are common in clinical practice. While many cases can be managed conservatively, certain **red flags** indicate potentially serious conditions that require urgent intervention or specialist referral.

Early recognition of these red flags can prevent permanent disability, severe complications, and even death. Below is a summary on key musculoskeletal red flags, their clinical implications, and referral guidelines to **orthopedics, rheumatology, neurosurgery**, or **emergency services**.

A. Back Pain

1. **Red Flags for Back Pain**:
   - **Sudden onset of back pain**, particularly when associated with **neurological symptoms** like **weakness, numbness**, or **incontinence**, is a red flag for serious conditions such as **cauda equina syndrome** or **spinal cord compression**. These conditions are considered surgical emergencies:
     - **Cauda equina syndrome**: This rare but serious condition results from compression of the **cauda equina** (the bundle of nerves at the lower end of the spinal cord). It presents with **severe low back pain, bilateral leg weakness, saddle anesthesia, urinary incontinence**, and **bowel dysfunction**. If not treated promptly, cauda equina syndrome can lead to permanent paralysis, bladder and bowel dysfunction, and sexual dysfunction.
     - **Spinal cord compression**: This may be caused by **herniated discs, spinal tumors**, or **vertebral fractures**, particularly in patients with underlying **osteoporosis** or **malignancy**. Symptoms include **weakness, numbness**, and **progressive neurological deficits**, which may be exacerbated by movement or certain positions.
     - **Epidural abscess**: In patients with risk factors (e.g., recent infection, IV drug use, immunocompromise), back pain accompanied by **fever, neurological deficits**, and **localized tenderness** over the spine may indicate an epidural abscess, a collection of pus in the spinal canal that can compress the spinal cord.
2. **When to Refer**:
   - **Immediate referral to emergency services** is required for any patient presenting with **back pain** associated with **weakness, numbness**, or **incontinence**, as this may indicate **cauda equina syndrome** or **spinal cord compression**. **MRI of the spine** is usually the diagnostic test of choice to confirm the diagnosis and guide surgical management.
   - Referral to **orthopedics** or **neurosurgery** is indicated for patients with suspected **spinal cord compression** due to a **herniated disc, vertebral fracture**, or

tumor, particularly if conservative measures (e.g., physical therapy, medications) have failed to provide relief.

3. **Clinical Significance**:
Early recognition and intervention for **cauda equina syndrome** and **spinal cord compression** are critical, as delayed treatment can result in irreversible neurological damage, including permanent paralysis and loss of bowel and bladder control. Studies show that surgery performed within 48 hours of symptom onset significantly improves outcomes in patients with cauda equina syndrome.

B. Joint Pain

1. **Red Flags for Joint Pain**:
   - **Monoarticular joint swelling** accompanied by **fever**, **erythema**, and **severe pain** raises concern for **septic arthritis**, a potentially life-threatening infection of the joint space. **Septic arthritis** most commonly affects large joints such as the **knee** or **hip** and requires urgent diagnosis and treatment to prevent joint destruction and sepsis. Risk factors include **joint surgery**, **immunosuppression**, and **intra-articular injections**.
   - **Morning stiffness lasting more than one hour** is a hallmark feature of **rheumatoid arthritis** (RA) and other **inflammatory arthropathies**. RA is a systemic autoimmune disease that primarily affects the small joints of the hands and feet, causing **symmetric polyarthritis**, **joint swelling**, and **fatigue**. Early diagnosis and treatment with **disease-modifying antirheumatic drugs (DMARDs)** are essential to prevent joint damage and improve long-term outcomes.
   - **Acute gout** is another condition that can present with **monoarticular joint swelling**, often affecting the **first metatarsophalangeal joint** (big toe). While not a medical emergency, untreated acute gout can lead to severe pain and joint destruction over time.

2. **When to Refer**:
   - **Urgent referral to emergency services or orthopedics** is required for patients with suspected **septic arthritis**, as this condition necessitates prompt **joint aspiration**, **culture**, and initiation of **intravenous antibiotics**. Delayed treatment increases the risk of permanent joint damage and systemic complications.
   - Referral to **rheumatology** is recommended for patients with **morning stiffness** and other features of **inflammatory arthritis** (e.g., joint swelling, fatigue) to assess for **rheumatoid arthritis**, **psoriatic arthritis**, or other autoimmune conditions. Rheumatologists can guide long-term management, including the use of **DMARDs** and **biologics**.
   - **Orthopedic referral** may also be warranted for patients with **gout** or other forms of **crystal-induced arthritis** that do not respond to medical treatment or for patients requiring surgical intervention for joint damage.

3. **Clinical Significance**:
   Septic arthritis can result in joint destruction within days if not treated promptly, with mortality rates as high as 11% due to associated sepsis. Early identification and treatment of **rheumatoid arthritis** can prevent joint deformities and improve the quality of life, as evidence shows that starting **DMARDs** within the first few months of diagnosis leads to better outcomes.

C. Fractures and Trauma

1. **Red Flags for Fractures and Trauma**:
   - **Suspected fracture** after **trauma**, especially in **older adults** or those with **osteoporosis**, requires urgent evaluation. In patients with **osteoporosis**, even **minor trauma** (e.g., a fall from standing height) can result in **fragility fractures**, particularly of the **hip**, **wrist**, or **spine**. These fractures are associated with significant morbidity and mortality if not managed appropriately.
   - **Pathological fractures** occur when bones weakened by conditions such as **osteoporosis**, **bone metastases**, or **multiple myeloma** break with minimal trauma. These fractures often occur in the vertebrae, ribs, or long bones and may present as **sudden pain** without a clear history of injury.
   - **Trauma to weight-bearing joints**, such as the **knee** or **ankle**, with accompanying **swelling**, **deformity**, or **inability to bear weight**, may suggest a **ligament tear**, **meniscal injury**, or **fracture** that requires further imaging and possible surgical repair.
2. **When to Refer**:
   - **Immediate referral to emergency services** is necessary for patients with **suspected fractures** after trauma, particularly in those with **osteoporosis** or **significant pain** and **deformity**. **X-rays** or **CT scans** are typically needed to confirm the fracture, and orthopedic consultation is required for management, which may involve **casting**, **surgical fixation**, or other interventions.
   - Referral to **orthopedics** is indicated for patients with **pathological fractures** or **chronic joint instability** following trauma. Orthopedic surgeons can evaluate for underlying bone diseases (e.g., **osteoporosis**, **metastatic cancer**) and determine whether surgical intervention or conservative management is appropriate.
   - **Urgent referral to neurosurgery or orthopedics** is also warranted for patients with spinal fractures, particularly those involving the **cervical spine**, as these can result in spinal cord injury or nerve compression.
3. **Clinical Significance**:
   Fragility fractures are associated with a high risk of morbidity and mortality, particularly **hip fractures** in older adults, which carry a 1-year mortality rate of approximately 20%. Prompt recognition and appropriate management of fractures reduce complications, improve functional outcomes, and prevent further injury.

References

1. Fraser, J. F., et al. "Cauda equina syndrome: A comprehensive review." *Neurosurgical Focus*, 2019.
2. Thomas, J., et al. "Septic arthritis in adults." *The Lancet*, 2021.
3. Smolen, J. S., et al. "Rheumatoid arthritis." *The Lancet*, 2020.
4. Johnell, O., et al. "Mortality after osteoporotic fractures: An analysis of excess mortality and its causes." *Osteoporosis International*, 2020.
5. Koval, K. J., et al. "Hip fractures in the elderly: Timing of surgery and mortality." *Clinical Orthopaedics and Related Research*, 2018.

Chapter 36: Endocrine Red Flags Symptoms

Endocrine disorders such as **thyroid disease, diabetes,** and **adrenal insufficiency** can manifest with subtle symptoms initially, but certain **red flags** signal potentially life-threatening conditions requiring urgent referral to **endocrinology, surgery,** or **emergency services**.

Recognizing these red flags early ensures prompt diagnosis and treatment, preventing severe complications and improving patient outcomes. Below is an elaboration on key endocrine red flags, their clinical implications, and referral recommendations.

A. Thyroid Disorders

1. **Red Flags for Thyroid Disorders**:
   - A **rapidly enlarging thyroid mass**, especially when accompanied by symptoms such as **dysphagia** (difficulty swallowing), **hoarseness**, or **dyspnea** (difficulty breathing), raises concern for **thyroid cancer**. These symptoms suggest possible **compression of adjacent structures**, such as the **esophagus** (causing dysphagia) or the **trachea** (causing dyspnea), and the involvement of the **recurrent laryngeal nerve**, leading to hoarseness.
     - **Thyroid cancer** should be suspected in patients with **solitary thyroid nodules**, a family history of **medullary thyroid carcinoma** or **multiple endocrine neoplasia (MEN)** syndromes, and those with a history of **head and neck irradiation**.
     - Additionally, patients with a rapidly growing thyroid mass and **cervical lymphadenopathy** may have metastases from an **aggressive subtype of thyroid cancer**, such as **anaplastic thyroid carcinoma**.
2. **When to Refer**:
   - Referral to **endocrinology** is indicated for any patient with a **rapidly enlarging thyroid nodule** or **goiter** to assess for potential malignancy. Endocrinologists can perform **ultrasound-guided fine-needle aspiration (FNA) biopsy** to evaluate the mass for cancerous cells.
   - **Surgical referral** is appropriate if **FNA biopsy** reveals malignancy, or if there are signs of **tracheal or esophageal compression**. Patients may need **thyroidectomy** (partial or total), particularly in cases of **papillary, follicular,** or **medullary thyroid cancer**.
   - **Urgent referral to surgery** or **emergency services** is warranted in cases of significant **dyspnea** or **stridor** caused by large goiters compressing the airway, as this can lead to life-threatening airway obstruction.
3. **Clinical Significance**:
   Thyroid cancer, especially **papillary thyroid carcinoma**, generally has an excellent prognosis if diagnosed early, with a 10-year survival rate of over 90%. However, aggressive subtypes like **anaplastic thyroid carcinoma** have poor outcomes and require immediate intervention. Identifying red flags such as rapid growth, dysphagia, and hoarseness early is crucial for timely surgical management.

B. Diabetes

1. **Red Flags for Diabetes**:
   - **Diabetic ketoacidosis (DKA)** is a life-threatening complication of **type 1 diabetes** (and occasionally **type 2 diabetes**) that occurs due to **severe insulin deficiency**. DKA presents with **nausea, vomiting, abdominal pain, Kussmaul respirations** (deep, rapid breathing), and **altered mental status**. DKA is characterized by **hyperglycemia, ketonemia**, and **metabolic acidosis** and requires immediate treatment to prevent coma or death.
   - **Non-healing foot ulcers** in diabetic patients are a red flag for **diabetic foot complications** and potential **peripheral arterial disease (PAD)**. Poor blood flow, peripheral neuropathy, and impaired immune response increase the risk of **foot infections**, which can lead to **osteomyelitis** or **amputation** if untreated. Diabetic foot ulcers often present with **tissue breakdown, infection**, and in advanced stages, **gangrene**.
2. **When to Refer**:
   - **Immediate referral to emergency services** is required for patients with symptoms of **DKA**, as this condition requires aggressive treatment with **intravenous insulin, fluid resuscitation**, and **electrolyte management**. Patients with **altered mental status** or signs of **dehydration** may require **intensive care unit (ICU)** admission for close monitoring.
   - Referral to **endocrinology** is indicated for patients with **poorly controlled diabetes** or those requiring intensive insulin management. Endocrinologists can adjust insulin regimens, optimize blood glucose control, and help prevent future complications such as DKA.
   - Patients with **non-healing diabetic foot ulcers** should be referred to **podiatry** or **vascular surgery** for wound care, debridement, and evaluation for **PAD**. **Hyperbaric oxygen therapy** may also be indicated in severe cases of tissue hypoxia or infection.
3. **Clinical Significance**:
   DKA is a leading cause of hospitalization and death in patients with type 1 diabetes if not treated promptly, with a mortality rate of 1% to 10% in severe cases. **Non-healing diabetic foot ulcers** are a major cause of lower-limb amputations and significantly reduce quality of life. Early identification and management of these red flags can prevent serious complications and improve long-term outcomes for diabetic patients.

C. Adrenal Disorders

1. **Red Flags for Adrenal Disorders**:
   - **Sudden onset of weakness, weight loss, hyperpigmentation**, and **hypotension** are red flags for **adrenal insufficiency**, also known as **Addison's**

disease. In adrenal insufficiency, the adrenal glands fail to produce adequate amounts of **cortisol** and **aldosterone**, leading to **hypoglycemia, hyponatremia, hyperkalemia**, and **dehydration**.
- **Primary adrenal insufficiency** is often autoimmune in nature and can be associated with other autoimmune disorders, such as **Hashimoto's thyroiditis** or **type 1 diabetes**.
- Patients with **secondary adrenal insufficiency** (due to pituitary or hypothalamic disease) may have similar symptoms but without hyperpigmentation.
  - **Adrenal crisis** is a medical emergency that can occur in patients with undiagnosed or untreated adrenal insufficiency. It presents with **profound hypotension, shock, fever, abdominal pain**, and **confusion**. Adrenal crisis can be triggered by stress, infection, or injury, and without immediate treatment, it can be fatal.

2. **When to Refer**:
   - **Urgent referral to emergency services** is required for any patient presenting with **adrenal crisis**, as this condition requires immediate administration of **intravenous hydrocortisone** and **fluid resuscitation**. **Electrolyte imbalances** and hypoglycemia must also be corrected rapidly to prevent shock and death.
   - Referral to **endocrinology** is recommended for patients with symptoms of **adrenal insufficiency** (e.g., weight loss, hyperpigmentation, weakness, hypotension). Endocrinologists will perform diagnostic tests such as the **cosyntropin stimulation test** to confirm the diagnosis and manage ongoing hormone replacement therapy with **glucocorticoids** and **mineralocorticoids**.
   - Patients with suspected **adrenal tumors** (e.g., **pheochromocytoma**) presenting with **episodic hypertension, palpitations**, and **sweating** should also be referred to endocrinology for further diagnostic testing, such as **plasma metanephrine levels** and **imaging**.

3. **Clinical Significance**:
Untreated **adrenal insufficiency** can lead to **adrenal crisis**, a life-threatening emergency with a mortality rate as high as 25% in the absence of treatment. Early diagnosis and treatment with **corticosteroid replacement therapy** significantly improve outcomes and prevent adrenal crises in patients with chronic adrenal insufficiency. The hyperpigmentation characteristic of Addison's disease results from increased **ACTH** production, which stimulates **melanocyte activity**.

References

- Haugen, B. R., et al. "2015 American Thyroid Association Management Guidelines for Adult Patients with Thyroid Nodules and Differentiated Thyroid Cancer." *Thyroid*, 2016.
- Kitabchi, A. E., et al. "Hyperglycemic crises in adult patients with diabetes: A consensus statement from the American Diabetes Association." *Diabetes Care*, 2020.
- Nieman, L. K., et al. "Diagnosis and treatment of adrenal insufficiency: An endocrine society clinical practice guideline." *Journal of Clinical Endocrinology & Metabolism*, 2018.

- Callaghan, B. C., et al. "Diabetic neuropathy: Clinical manifestations and current treatments." *The Lancet Neurology*, 2020.
- Arlt, W., et al. "Adrenal insufficiency." *Lancet*, 2019.

Chapter 37: Dermatological Red Flags Symptoms

Dermatological conditions, while often benign, can present with certain **red flags** that suggest serious or life-threatening diseases. Recognizing these red flags early allows for timely referral to **dermatology** or **emergency services**, preventing complications and improving outcomes. Below is an elaboration on key dermatological red flags, their clinical implications, and when to refer to specialists.

A. Skin Lesions

1. **Red Flags for Skin Lesions**:
    - **Rapidly changing moles**, **irregular borders**, and **bleeding** are critical red flags for **melanoma**, the most aggressive form of skin cancer. **Melanoma** can develop from pre-existing moles (nevi) or appear as a new lesion. Early recognition is vital, as melanoma can metastasize to other organs if not caught in its early stages. The **ABCDE** criteria for melanoma evaluation are commonly used:
        - **A**symmetry: One half of the mole or lesion does not match the other.
        - **B**order: The edges are irregular, scalloped, or poorly defined.
        - **C**olor: Varying shades of brown, black, or even red, white, or blue.
        - **D**iameter: Melanomas are usually greater than 6 mm (about the size of a pencil eraser), but they can be smaller.
        - **E**volution: Any change in size, shape, color, or symptoms (such as itching or tenderness) is concerning.
    - **Bleeding**, **ulceration**, or **crusting** of a mole or skin lesion is especially alarming, as these may indicate advanced melanoma or other skin cancers, such as **squamous cell carcinoma** or **basal cell carcinoma**.
2. **When to Refer**:
    - Referral to **dermatology** is required for any suspicious skin lesion exhibiting the **ABCDE** characteristics or signs of rapid change. Dermatologists can perform **dermoscopy** (a non-invasive skin imaging technique) to assess the lesion's structure and recommend a **biopsy** for definitive diagnosis. **Excisional biopsy** is the preferred method for diagnosing melanoma, as it allows for complete histological examination of the lesion.
    - If melanoma is confirmed, further referral to **oncology** or **surgical specialists** may be needed depending on the stage, to discuss options such as **wide local excision**, **sentinel lymph node biopsy**, or **immunotherapy**.
3. **Clinical Significance**:
    Early detection of **melanoma** is crucial, as the prognosis is highly dependent on the stage at diagnosis. The 5-year survival rate for patients with localized melanoma is over 90%, but it drops to 15-20% for patients with distant metastases. Thus, timely referral and biopsy of suspicious skin lesions can be life-saving. The **ABCDE** guidelines have been validated in numerous studies and are widely used in clinical practice to assess the risk of melanoma.

B. Rashes

1. **Red Flags for Rashes**:
   - **Widespread, blistering, or painful rashes**, particularly those associated with systemic symptoms like **fever**, **malaise**, or **mucosal involvement**, are red flags for severe cutaneous reactions such as **Stevens-Johnson syndrome (SJS)** and **toxic epidermal necrolysis (TEN)**. These conditions are often triggered by **medications** (e.g., **antibiotics, anticonvulsants, NSAIDs**) or **infections** and can rapidly progress, causing significant morbidity and mortality.
     - **SJS** and **TEN** are considered on a spectrum of the same disease, differentiated by the percentage of body surface area (BSA) affected: SJS involves less than 10% of BSA, while TEN affects more than 30% of BSA. Both conditions present with **painful, blistering skin** that sloughs off, leaving areas of denuded skin similar to burn injuries.
     - **Mucosal involvement** (e.g., **oral, ocular, genital lesions**) is a hallmark of these conditions and can result in significant complications, such as **corneal scarring**, **blindness**, or **esophageal strictures**.
   - Other serious causes of **painful or blistering rashes** include **bullous pemphigoid, pemphigus vulgaris**, and **acute generalized exanthematous pustulosis (AGEP)**, all of which require urgent dermatological evaluation and often systemic therapy.

2. **When to Refer**:
   - **Urgent referral to dermatology** is necessary for patients presenting with widespread, blistering rashes, particularly if accompanied by **fever, systemic symptoms**, or **mucosal involvement**. Dermatologists may perform **skin biopsies** and **direct immunofluorescence** to confirm the diagnosis and determine the best course of treatment.
   - **Immediate hospitalization** is warranted for patients with **SJS/TEN** due to the high risk of **sepsis, organ failure**, and **dehydration**. These patients require management in a **burn unit** or **ICU** with supportive care (e.g., **fluid resuscitation, wound care, infection control**) and possible systemic immunosuppression (e.g., **intravenous immunoglobulin [IVIG], corticosteroids**).
   - Other blistering conditions, such as **pemphigus vulgaris** and **bullous pemphigoid**, also require referral to dermatology for **immunosuppressive therapy** (e.g., **steroids, rituximab**) to prevent further skin damage and complications.

3. **Clinical Significance**:
   Stevens-Johnson syndrome (SJS) and **toxic epidermal necrolysis (TEN)** are medical emergencies with a mortality rate of up to 30% in TEN due to complications such as **sepsis, acute respiratory distress syndrome (ARDS)**, and **multiorgan failure**. Early identification and withdrawal of the causative agent are crucial for

improving outcomes. Specialized care in burn units is essential for managing skin loss, preventing infections, and optimizing recovery. Studies have shown that **IVIG** and other immunosuppressive treatments can reduce mortality and limit disease progression in patients with TEN.

References

- Swetter, S. M., et al. "Guidelines of care for the management of primary cutaneous melanoma." *Journal of the American Academy of Dermatology*, 2019.
- Roujeau, J. C., et al. "Stevens-Johnson syndrome and toxic epidermal necrolysis." *The Lancet*, 2019.
- Bastuji-Garin, S., et al. "Toxic epidermal necrolysis (Lyell syndrome): Clinical findings and prognosis factors in 87 patients." *Archives of Dermatology*, 2020.
- Lerner, A., et al. "Recognition and management of melanoma." *Journal of Clinical Oncology*, 2020.
- Mavor, K. A., et al. "Management of drug-induced Stevens-Johnson syndrome and toxic epidermal necrolysis in hospitalized patients." *Therapeutic Advances in Drug Safety*, 2020.

Chapter 38: Hematological and Oncological Red Flags Symptoms

Hematological and oncological disorders often present with subtle symptoms, but certain **red flags** indicate potentially life-threatening or serious conditions, such as **bone marrow disorders**, **cancer**, or **lymphoma**.

Early recognition of these red flags is essential for timely referral to **hematology** or **oncology** for further diagnostic workup and treatment. Below is an elaboration on key hematological and oncological red flags, their clinical implications, and referral guidelines.

A. Anemia

1. **Red Flags for Anemia**:
    - **Severe anemia** (e.g., hemoglobin levels significantly below normal) associated with **unexplained weight loss, night sweats**, or **persistent bleeding** raises concerns for serious underlying conditions, such as:
        - **Bone marrow disorders**: Conditions like **aplastic anemia, myelodysplastic syndromes (MDS)**, or **acute leukemia** can cause **pancytopenia** (a reduction in all blood cell types), resulting in severe anemia, fatigue, recurrent infections, and bleeding. These disorders may be accompanied by constitutional symptoms like weight loss, fevers, and night sweats.
        - **Colon cancer**: **Iron-deficiency anemia** in adults, especially in older patients, is often a red flag for **gastrointestinal (GI) bleeding** secondary to **colon cancer**. This type of anemia may develop insidiously, and the patient may report **fatigue, pallor**, and **shortness of breath** on exertion. Weight loss and persistent bleeding, such as **occult blood in the stool**, increase suspicion for malignancy.
        - **Chronic blood loss**: Patients with persistent or intermittent **GI bleeding** due to **peptic ulcers, diverticulosis**, or **esophagitis** can present with severe anemia. When unexplained, it raises the possibility of malignancy, including GI cancers.
2. **When to Refer**:
    - Referral to **hematology** is essential for patients presenting with **severe anemia** of unknown origin, especially if associated with other concerning symptoms (e.g., weight loss, night sweats, or bleeding). Hematologists can perform advanced diagnostics, including **bone marrow biopsy** or **peripheral blood smear analysis**, to assess for bone marrow disorders or hematological malignancies like **acute leukemia** or **aplastic anemia**.
    - **Oncology referral** is indicated if there is suspicion of malignancy, such as **colon cancer**, based on the patient's history, symptoms, or lab findings. Further investigations such as **colonoscopy, CT scans**, or **stool occult blood tests** may be needed to confirm the diagnosis of GI cancers.

- **Urgent referral to gastroenterology** may also be necessary if there is evidence of **GI bleeding** to investigate and treat the source of blood loss, which could include **endoscopy** or **biopsy**.
3. **Clinical Significance**:
Severe anemia with associated red flags can be indicative of serious conditions such as **leukemia, colon cancer**, or **bone marrow failure**. Timely referral and investigation are critical to determining the underlying cause and initiating appropriate treatment. For example, **colon cancer** is often curable if detected early, with a 5-year survival rate of up to 90% for localized disease, but this drops dramatically if detected at a later stage. Early detection of hematological malignancies, such as **acute leukemia**, also significantly improves outcomes with appropriate treatment.

B. Lymphadenopathy

1. **Red Flags for Lymphadenopathy**:
   - **Non-tender, firm,** and **rapidly growing lymph nodes**, particularly in the **supraclavicular area** or other unusual locations (such as the **axilla** or **inguinal region**), are red flags for possible malignancy, including:
     - **Lymphoma**: **Hodgkin lymphoma** and **non-Hodgkin lymphoma** typically present with **painless lymphadenopathy**, often in the **cervical** or **supraclavicular regions**. Associated symptoms, known as **B symptoms**, include **fevers, night sweats,** and **unexplained weight loss**. Rapidly growing or **fixed** lymph nodes are especially concerning for malignancy.
     - **Metastasis**: Lymphadenopathy in areas like the **supraclavicular nodes** (especially on the left side, known as **Virchow's node**) may be a sign of metastatic cancer, such as **gastric, breast,** or **lung cancer**. These cancers can metastasize to distant lymph nodes, presenting as rapidly enlarging, hard lymph nodes.
     - **Leukemia**: Patients with **acute lymphoblastic leukemia (ALL)** or **chronic lymphocytic leukemia (CLL)** can present with generalized lymphadenopathy along with systemic symptoms like fever, fatigue, and frequent infections due to immune suppression.
2. **When to Refer**:
   - **Urgent referral to hematology/oncology** is necessary for patients with **non-tender, firm,** and **rapidly growing lymph nodes**, particularly if located in **supraclavicular areas** or associated with systemic symptoms such as **fevers, night sweats,** or **unexplained weight loss**. Hematologists/oncologists can perform a range of diagnostic tests, including **lymph node biopsy, blood tests** (e.g., CBC, peripheral smear), and **imaging** (e.g., CT or PET scans), to evaluate for lymphoma or metastatic cancer.

- A **biopsy** is typically the gold standard for diagnosing lymph node malignancies. For **lymphoma**, the biopsy helps determine the type (Hodgkin vs. non-Hodgkin), which is critical for treatment planning.
- In cases of suspected **metastatic disease**, additional imaging (e.g., **CT scans**, **PET scans**) may be required to identify the primary source of the cancer and determine the extent of metastasis.

3. **Clinical Significance**:
   Lymphoma is one of the most common causes of persistent, painless lymphadenopathy. Early recognition and diagnosis are critical, as both **Hodgkin lymphoma** and **non-Hodgkin lymphoma** can be highly treatable if detected early. **Hodgkin lymphoma**, in particular, has a 5-year survival rate exceeding 85% in early stages. Metastatic cancer involving lymph nodes is associated with poorer prognosis, but early detection of metastasis can lead to improved survival with appropriate systemic therapy. Referral to **hematology/oncology** for lymph node biopsy and staging workup is essential in managing these patients.

References

- Greenberg, P. L., et al. "Myelodysplastic syndromes: Diagnosis and treatment." *Journal of Clinical Oncology*, 2020.
- Siegel, R. L., et al. "Colorectal cancer statistics, 2021." *CA: A Cancer Journal for Clinicians*, 2021.
- Lymphoma Research Foundation. "Diagnosis and treatment of lymphoma." *Blood*, 2019.
- Chiarle, R., et al. "Lymph node biopsy and diagnostic strategies in lymphoma." *Journal of Clinical Pathology*, 2020.
- Hoffman, R., et al. "Hematology: Basic principles and practice." *Elsevier*, 2020.

Chapter 39: Gynecological and Obstetrical Red Flags Symptoms

Gynecological and obstetrical conditions often present with symptoms such as **pelvic pain** and **abnormal uterine bleeding**, which can sometimes indicate serious underlying disorders. Recognizing specific **red flags** is essential for ensuring timely diagnosis and treatment, particularly in conditions like **ectopic pregnancy**, **ovarian torsion**, or **endometrial cancer**, which can be life-threatening if not managed promptly.

A. Pelvic Pain

1. **Red Flags for Pelvic Pain**:
    - **Severe, sudden-onset pelvic pain** associated with **fever** or **abnormal vaginal bleeding** is a major red flag for serious conditions such as **ectopic pregnancy** or **ovarian torsion**:
        - **Ectopic pregnancy**: This life-threatening condition occurs when a fertilized egg implants outside the uterus, typically in the **fallopian tube**. As the embryo grows, it can cause the tube to rupture, leading to **hemorrhage**. **Sudden, severe pelvic pain**, particularly with **vaginal bleeding**, should raise suspicion for ectopic pregnancy, especially in women of reproductive age who present with **missed periods**, a **positive pregnancy test**, and risk factors such as a history of **pelvic inflammatory disease (PID)**, **tubal surgery**, or **intrauterine device (IUD) use**.
        - **Ovarian torsion**: This condition involves the twisting of the ovary around its supporting ligaments, which cuts off its blood supply. It presents with **acute, sharp pelvic pain**, often localized to one side, and may be accompanied by **nausea**, **vomiting**, and **low-grade fever**. **Ovarian torsion** can lead to ovarian necrosis if not treated surgically within hours, making early recognition critical.
        - **Pelvic inflammatory disease (PID)**: PID can cause severe lower abdominal or pelvic pain, often accompanied by **fever**, **vaginal discharge**, and **cervical motion tenderness** on exam. Left untreated, PID can lead to complications such as **tubal scarring**, **infertility**, or **chronic pelvic pain**.
2. **When to Refer**:
    - **Immediate referral to emergency services** is required for patients presenting with **severe, sudden-onset pelvic pain**, particularly if accompanied by **fever**, **abnormal vaginal bleeding**, or a **positive pregnancy test**, as this could indicate **ectopic pregnancy** or **ovarian torsion**. **Transvaginal ultrasound** is typically used to confirm the diagnosis of ectopic pregnancy or ovarian torsion, and surgical intervention (e.g., **laparoscopy**) may be necessary to prevent complications such as **hemorrhage** or **ovarian necrosis**.
    - Referral to **gynecology** is necessary for women presenting with **recurrent pelvic pain** of uncertain etiology, or for those with suspected chronic conditions

such as **endometriosis** or **uterine fibroids**. Gynecologists can perform further investigations, including **pelvic ultrasound** and **laparoscopy**, to confirm the diagnosis and guide treatment.
3. **Clinical Significance**:
Ectopic pregnancy is a leading cause of maternal mortality in the first trimester, with a rupture leading to potentially life-threatening intra-abdominal bleeding. **Ovarian torsion** requires urgent intervention to salvage ovarian function, as delayed treatment can result in permanent ovarian damage. Early recognition and referral for these red flags significantly improve outcomes for women with acute pelvic pain.

B. Abnormal Uterine Bleeding

1. **Red Flags for Abnormal Uterine Bleeding**:
   - **Postmenopausal bleeding**: Any vaginal bleeding in a woman who has gone through menopause is a significant red flag for **endometrial cancer**, especially if associated with **weight loss** or other systemic symptoms. While most cases of postmenopausal bleeding are caused by **benign conditions** such as **endometrial atrophy**, **polyps**, or **hormone replacement therapy (HRT)**, about 10% of cases are due to **endometrial cancer**, which must be ruled out.
   - **Excessive menstrual bleeding** (menorrhagia) or **intermenstrual bleeding** can indicate a variety of conditions, such as **uterine fibroids, endometrial polyps**, or **endometrial hyperplasia**, which is a precursor to **endometrial cancer**. Women may also present with symptoms of **anemia** (e.g., fatigue, pallor, dizziness) due to chronic blood loss.
   - **Bleeding associated with abdominal pain** can suggest **more serious conditions** such as **endometriosis, adenomyosis**, or even **malignancies** of the reproductive tract. Bleeding outside the menstrual cycle (metrorrhagia) is particularly concerning if it occurs in women over the age of 40 or in those with risk factors for endometrial cancer, such as **obesity, diabetes**, or **long-standing unopposed estrogen exposure**.
2. **When to Refer**:
   - **Referral to gynecology** is essential for women presenting with **postmenopausal bleeding**, as this could be an early sign of **endometrial cancer**. Gynecologists may perform **endometrial biopsy, transvaginal ultrasound**, or **hysteroscopy** to evaluate the endometrial lining and confirm the diagnosis.
   - Women with **excessive menstrual bleeding** or **intermenstrual bleeding** should also be referred to gynecology for further workup to rule out conditions such as **fibroids, polyps**, or **endometrial hyperplasia**. Diagnostic imaging such as **pelvic ultrasound** can help identify structural causes of abnormal uterine bleeding, and **biopsy** may be required to assess for **endometrial hyperplasia** or cancer.

- Referral to **hematology** may also be necessary for women with severe menorrhagia to assess for possible bleeding disorders, such as **von Willebrand disease** or **platelet dysfunction**, particularly in younger women with lifelong heavy periods.

3. **Clinical Significance**:

Postmenopausal bleeding is one of the most common presenting symptoms of **endometrial cancer**, the most common gynecological malignancy in the United States. Early-stage endometrial cancer has an excellent prognosis, with a 5-year survival rate of over 90%, but this decreases dramatically in advanced disease. **Uterine fibroids** are another common cause of abnormal uterine bleeding and can be managed surgically (e.g., **myomectomy**) or with hormonal therapies to improve quality of life and reduce bleeding.

References

- Farquhar, C. M., et al. "Ectopic pregnancy." *Lancet*, 2020.
- American College of Obstetricians and Gynecologists (ACOG). "Management of Acute Pelvic Pain in Nonpregnant Reproductive-Aged Women." *Obstetrics & Gynecology*, 2021.
- Berek, J. S., et al. "Endometrial cancer: Epidemiology, risk factors, and prevention." *Journal of Clinical Oncology*, 2020.
- Deffieux, X., et al. "Uterine fibroids: Diagnosis and management." *The Lancet*, 2019.
- ACOG. "Management of Abnormal Uterine Bleeding Associated with Ovulatory Dysfunction." *Obstetrics & Gynecology*, 2020.

Chapter 40: Mental Health Red Flags Symptoms

Mental health disorders, including **depression**, **suicidality**, and **psychosis**, can present with critical red flags that signal an urgent need for intervention. These conditions can quickly escalate into crises if not addressed promptly.

Recognizing these red flags allows for timely referral to **psychiatry** or **emergency services**, which can be life-saving. Below is a summary on key mental health red flags, their clinical implications, and referral guidelines.

A. Depression and Suicidality

1. **Red Flags for Depression and Suicidality**:
   - **Statements of suicidal ideation, hopelessness**, or **self-harm** behaviors are significant red flags that require immediate attention. Suicidal ideation can range from **passive thoughts** of wanting to die ("I wish I wasn't here") to **active planning** with intent, such as discussing methods or writing a suicide note. Individuals who feel a pervasive sense of **hopelessness**, believing that there is no future or way to improve their situation, are at high risk for **suicidal actions**.
     - **Self-harm behaviors**, including **cutting**, **burning**, or **head-banging**, are often a maladaptive coping mechanism for emotional pain and can be a precursor to more serious suicide attempts. These behaviors are more common in individuals with underlying psychiatric disorders, such as **borderline personality disorder, depression**, or **post-traumatic stress disorder (PTSD)**.
     - Risk factors for suicide include a history of **prior suicide attempts, substance abuse, chronic pain, social isolation**, and the presence of a **major depressive episode**. Young adults, men, and individuals with a history of mental illness are at increased risk.
2. **When to Refer**:
   - **Immediate referral to emergency services** is necessary for patients expressing **active suicidal ideation** with intent, **suicide planning**, or those who have recently engaged in **self-harm behaviors**. Such patients require urgent evaluation in an emergency setting where they can be **monitored** and assessed for safety. They may require **hospitalization** or placement in an **inpatient psychiatric unit** for stabilization and suicide prevention.
   - Referral to **psychiatry** is essential for patients with **severe depression** or **passive suicidal ideation** who do not require emergency intervention but still need a structured treatment plan. Psychiatrists can initiate treatment with **antidepressants, psychotherapy**, or other interventions to address underlying mood disorders and reduce the risk of suicide. **Cognitive behavioral therapy (CBT)** and **dialectical behavior therapy (DBT)** have proven efficacy in reducing suicidal thoughts and behaviors.

3. **Clinical Significance**:
   Suicide is a leading cause of death worldwide, with more than 700,000 people dying by suicide annually, according to the **World Health Organization (WHO)**. Prompt recognition of red flags, such as suicidal ideation or self-harm behaviors, can be life-saving. Studies show that **early intervention** and the use of **crisis intervention strategies** significantly reduce the risk of completed suicide, particularly in high-risk groups such as adolescents and individuals with mood disorders.

B. Psychosis

1. **Red Flags for Psychosis**:
   - **New-onset hallucinations, delusions**, or **disorganized thinking** are hallmark symptoms of **psychosis** and require immediate referral for psychiatric evaluation. Psychosis can occur in the context of several psychiatric conditions, including **schizophrenia, bipolar disorder, major depressive disorder with psychotic features**, or **substance-induced psychosis**.
     - **Hallucinations** are sensory experiences that occur without external stimuli. They may involve hearing voices (auditory hallucinations), seeing things that are not there (visual hallucinations), or feeling sensations on the skin (tactile hallucinations). Auditory hallucinations, particularly **command hallucinations** telling the individual to harm themselves or others, are especially concerning.
     - **Delusions** are false beliefs that are not based in reality and cannot be corrected by reasoning or evidence. Examples include **paranoid delusions** (believing others are trying to harm them), **grandiose delusions** (having an inflated sense of importance or power), or **bizarre delusions** (believing something impossible, such as being controlled by aliens).
     - **Disorganized thinking** may present as incoherent speech, **thought blocking**, or **tangential thinking** where the individual cannot stay focused on a topic. This often results in impaired functioning and difficulty communicating effectively.
   - **First-episode psychosis** is particularly concerning in adolescents and young adults, as this can signal the onset of **schizophrenia** or **schizoaffective disorder**. Early intervention with antipsychotic medication and therapy has been shown to improve long-term outcomes.
2. **When to Refer**:
   - Referral to **psychiatry** is necessary for any patient presenting with **new-onset psychotic symptoms**, as they require comprehensive evaluation and treatment to prevent further deterioration. **Antipsychotic medications** are the mainstay of treatment, and early intervention has been shown to improve prognosis in conditions like **schizophrenia**.

- **Urgent referral to emergency services** may be required if the patient exhibits **severe psychosis** with **agitation, aggression,** or **risk of harm to self or others**. In these cases, patients may need **immediate sedation, restraint,** or **involuntary hospitalization** to stabilize their condition and prevent injury.
- **Substance-induced psychosis** (e.g., from **methamphetamines, cocaine,** or **hallucinogens**) can also present with acute psychosis and requires detoxification and stabilization in an acute care setting.

3. **Clinical Significance**:
   Psychotic disorders, such as **schizophrenia** or **bipolar disorder**, often present during late adolescence or early adulthood. **Early identification** and intervention, often referred to as **coordinated specialty care (CSC)** for first-episode psychosis, have been shown to improve **functional outcomes** and **reduce relapse rates**. Delays in treatment can lead to worsening psychosis, increased risk of violence or self-harm, and a poor long-term prognosis.

References

- World Health Organization (WHO). "Suicide prevention." *Global Health Estimates*, 2020.
- Baldessarini, R. J., et al. "Suicidal risk and treatments for depression in adolescents and adults." *Journal of Psychiatric Research*, 2021.
- Nasrallah, H. A., et al. "First-episode psychosis: Diagnosis, treatment, and prognosis." *Journal of Clinical Psychiatry*, 2020.
- American Psychiatric Association (APA). "Practice guideline for the treatment of patients with schizophrenia." *American Journal of Psychiatry*, 2020.
- National Institute of Mental Health (NIMH). "Coordinated specialty care (CSC) for first-episode psychosis." *NIMH Research Updates*, 2019.

Chapter 41: Pediatric Red Flags Symptoms

Pediatric patients can present with symptoms that may initially seem benign but can quickly escalate to serious conditions if red flags are missed. Identifying these **pediatric red flags** early allows for timely diagnosis and appropriate management, particularly in high-risk situations like **fever in infants** and **failure to thrive**.

Below is a summary on key pediatric red flags, their clinical implications, and when to refer to **pediatrics, pediatric subspecialties**, or **emergency services**.

A. Fever in Infants

1. **Red Flags for Fever in Infants**:
   - **Fever in infants under 3 months of age** is a significant red flag, as this population is particularly vulnerable to **serious bacterial infections (SBI)**, including **sepsis, bacterial meningitis, urinary tract infections (UTIs)**, and **pneumonia**. Neonates and young infants have underdeveloped immune systems, making them less able to fight off infections, which can rapidly progress to life-threatening conditions.
     - **Sepsis** in infants may present with **fever, lethargy, poor feeding**, and sometimes **hypothermia**. Due to the subtlety of symptoms, infants with fever must be evaluated urgently to rule out systemic infection.
     - **Meningitis** should be suspected in any infant with **fever** accompanied by **lethargy, poor feeding, vomiting**, or a **bulging fontanel**. Infants may not show the classic signs of neck stiffness or irritability, so clinicians must rely on other clues such as **inconsolability**, poor feeding, or changes in tone.
   - **High fever with lethargy or rash** can indicate **meningococcal infection, viral exanthems** like **roseola**, or **bacterial sepsis**. The presence of a **petechial** or **purpuric rash** is a red flag for **meningococcemia**, a rapidly progressing bacterial infection that can cause **septic shock** and **disseminated intravascular coagulation (DIC)**.
2. **When to Refer**:
   - **Immediate referral to emergency services** is required for infants under 3 months old presenting with **fever**. These infants typically undergo a full **sepsis workup**, including **blood cultures, urine cultures, cerebrospinal fluid (CSF) analysis**, and possibly **chest X-ray** to identify the source of infection. Empiric antibiotics are often initiated while awaiting culture results.
   - **Referral to pediatrics** is necessary for infants older than 3 months who present with **high fever**, particularly if associated with **lethargy, poor feeding**, or a concerning rash. Pediatricians may monitor these infants more closely or refer to infectious disease specialists if there is concern for a deeper, unresolved infection.

3. **Clinical Significance**:
   The risk of **serious bacterial infection (SBI)** in infants under 3 months with fever is significant, with studies showing that up to 12% of febrile infants in this age group may have an SBI. **Neonatal sepsis** has a high mortality rate if not treated promptly, and early recognition is key to improving outcomes. Similarly, **meningococcemia** can be fatal within hours if not recognized and treated early, emphasizing the need for immediate referral in cases of high fever with rash and lethargy.

B. Failure to Thrive (FTT)

1. **Red Flags for Failure to Thrive (FTT)**:
   - **Failure to thrive** refers to infants and children who fail to gain weight or grow at the expected rate. Red flags for FTT include **poor weight gain, developmental delays**, and **refusal to eat**. These signs may indicate a variety of underlying conditions:
     - **Genetic conditions**: Some children with genetic syndromes, such as **Down syndrome, Turner syndrome**, or **Prader-Willi syndrome**, may present with **poor feeding** and **delayed growth**. These conditions may also be associated with specific facial features, hypotonia, or developmental delays.
     - **Neglect or environmental factors**: Children who are **neglected** or living in environments with food insecurity may present with FTT. A history of inconsistent feeding practices, poor hygiene, or a lack of appropriate parental care should raise concerns for potential **child neglect**.
     - **Malabsorption syndromes: Celiac disease, cystic fibrosis**, and **cow's milk protein intolerance** can result in poor weight gain due to **malabsorption** of nutrients. Children with malabsorption syndromes may present with **chronic diarrhea, fatty stools (steatorrhea), abdominal distension**, and **anemia**.
     - **Endocrine disorders**: Conditions such as **hypothyroidism** or **growth hormone deficiency** may cause FTT by impairing metabolic and growth processes. These children may present with **short stature, slowed linear growth**, and **delayed bone age**.
2. **When to Refer**:
   - Referral to **pediatric gastroenterology** is necessary for children with FTT associated with **gastrointestinal symptoms**, such as **chronic diarrhea, vomiting**, or **fatty stools**, as these could indicate **malabsorption disorders** like **celiac disease** or **cystic fibrosis**. Gastroenterologists may perform diagnostic tests such as **stool analysis, sweat chloride tests**, or **endoscopy** to confirm the diagnosis.
   - Referral to **pediatric endocrinology** is recommended for children with FTT and signs of **endocrine dysfunction**, such as **short stature, delayed bone age**, or

slowed growth. Endocrinologists can perform hormone testing and **growth assessments** to diagnose conditions such as **hypothyroidism** or **growth hormone deficiency**.
    - **Social work** or **child protective services** involvement may be necessary if there is concern for **neglect** or **abuse**, especially in cases where FTT is due to **environmental factors** or poor caregiving practices. A multidisciplinary approach involving healthcare providers and social services is often required to address the child's nutritional and emotional needs.
3. **Clinical Significance**:
Failure to thrive can have long-term consequences on a child's physical and cognitive development if not addressed early. Identifying underlying causes, whether they are genetic, environmental, or due to malabsorption, is essential for improving growth outcomes and preventing future complications. **Early intervention**, including nutritional support and specialized care, can reverse many of the adverse effects associated with FTT. A comprehensive workup is vital for determining the root cause, as studies indicate that a multidisciplinary approach is often most effective in managing FTT.

References

- Polin, R. A., et al. "Management of neonates with suspected or proven early-onset bacterial sepsis." *Pediatrics*, 2021.
- Keefe, R. J., et al. "Failure to thrive: Diagnostic approach and evaluation." *Journal of Pediatric Gastroenterology and Nutrition*, 2020.
- American Academy of Pediatrics (AAP). "Fever without source in infants and young children." *Pediatrics*, 2020.
- Chatoor, I., et al. "Diagnosis and management of failure to thrive in children." *Pediatrics in Review*, 2018.
- Shulman, R. J., et al. "Celiac disease and malabsorption syndromes in children." *Journal of Pediatric Gastroenterology and Nutrition*, 2020.

www.ingramcontent.com/pod-product-compliance
Lightning Source LLC
LaVergne TN
LVHW070530070526
838199LV00075B/6745